THE COMPLETE MRCPSYCH
PART II

THE COMPLETE MRCPSYCH
PART II

ASHOK G. PATEL

MRCPsych, DPM
Consultant Psychiatrist,
Fairfield Hospital,
Hitchin, Hertfordshire

WB SAUNDERS COMPANY LTD
LONDON   PHILADELPHIA   TORONTO
SYDNEY   TOKYO

W. B. Saunders Company Ltd 24–28 Oval Road
London NW1 7DX, UK

The Curtis Center
Independence Square West
Philadelphia, PA 19106-3399
USA

Harcourt Brace & Company,
55 Horner Avenue
Toronto, Ontario M8Z 4X6
Canada

Harcourt Brace & Company,
Australia
30–52 Smidmore Street
Marrickville, NSW 2204
Australia

Harcourt Brace & Company,
Japan Inc.
Ichibancho Central Building
22-1 Ichibancho
Chiyoda-ku, Tokyo 102, Japan

A catalogue record for this book is available from the
British Library

ISBN 0–7020–1808–2

This book is printed on acid-free paper

Typeset by Paston Press Ltd, Loddon, Norfolk
Printed in Great Britain by Mackays of Chatham PLC,
Chatham, Kent

CONTENTS

PMPs ORAL EXAMINATION 183

FOREWORD

Dr Patel has written a book that will be eagerly read by candidates for the examination for Membership of the Royal College of Psychiatrists. His earlier publications on Multiple Choice Questions (MCQs) have been well received, and there is clearly a need for a volume that deals not only with MCQs, but also with other parts of the examination.

I have known Dr Patel for many years and he has an impressive track record. He was active in research before obtaining his post as Consultant Psychiatrist. Since then he has continued his interest in research and has published works of interest for physicians who wish to specialize in psychiatry. This would not be surprising if he were working full time in a university hospital or a medical school, but Dr Patel does not work in an ivory tower, but in a busy clinical department with the National Health Service. As a consultant in a typical psychiatric unit, he is able to see the requirements of the representative registrar or trainee in psychiatry, and to write in a way that is immediate and acceptable to such a junior doctor.

He is experienced not only in teaching and supervising medical practitioners who are training in psychiatry, but also in acting as an examiner for the Royal College of Psychiatrists. He is therefore able to assess the problems that candidates have when they come to take the examination. He knows what they find easy and what they find difficult and has been able to prepare the material in this book and present it in a way that meets their needs.

Although the College is not yet twenty-five years old, it has changed the format of the examination during that time, and there has been a dearth of books that are designed for the postgraduate student who wishes to practise each part of the examination.

In my own experience as an examiner I too have been struck by the fact that candidates do not always make full use of the knowledge that they do possess. For instance, in oral examinations the candidate will sometimes sit silent for a time, possibly trying to think of the best answer to a question. This is not a good policy since the candidate is not scoring any marks during the time that silence reigns. A better method usually is to give an approximate answer initially, and then to refine it, but to remain talking all the time. There is one proviso: the talking should be of a sort that reveals knowledge, rather than just waffling to fill in space.

The following example may illustrate this. If the candidate is told "Give me a delusion that is pathognomonic of schizophrenia" and for the moment cannot instantly recall an example, I would suggest the following answer, playing for time but revealing knowledge all the while. "While delusions may occur in any of the major psychoses, functional or organic, those that occur in schizophrenia are typically non-understandable or incongruous. That is to say, they cannot readily be understood as being secondary to an underlying mood state of depression or elation." Then (as recollection dawns) "Ah, yes, *primary* delusions are characteristic of schizophrenia." Alternatively, the candidate's ruminations to play for time may dwell on the bizarre quality of typical schizophrenic delusions, which then calls to mind the magical quality of the delusions grouped together as disorders of the possession of thought (thought broadcasting, thought removal, thought insertion). Generally, the thoughts going through the candidate's mind are worth sharing, worthy of some marks, and certainly better than the alternative – silence.

The other reason for not keeping silent is less obvious, unless one has in fact acted as an examiner. If a candidate is talking too much, or continuing for too long on a particular point, it is fairly easy for the examiner to indicate that he wishes to interrupt. The situation is more difficult with the silent candidate. The examiner may be afraid to intervene in the silence with helpful hints, unless these merely interrupt the candidate's train of thought, thus raising the anxiety level even further. Thus I believe that it is better for the candidate to try to say *something* rather than nothing at all.

All of us have taken many examinations before. It is easy to recall why sometimes silence seems to be temptingly golden. We are afraid of saying something wrong which, at worst, might make us fail the examination. Although we can readily understand this motivation, it is not a valid reason for keeping quiet. Experience shows that candidates are much more likely to do worse than they deserve because of reticence than because of making the occasional error. In particular, candidates can be reassured that it is possible to make mistakes and errors in examinations (even oral and clinical examinations) and still pass. I have done it myself.

Let us accept then that candidates would often do better if they concentrated positively on scoring marks and on revealing their knowledge, than on defensively avoiding any possibility of an error. I have illustrated this by describing the situation in an oral examination, but it is also true of the other parts of the examination that are covered in this book. It is even true of the MCQs. Here I would suggest that in rehearsing for the examination readers attempt an MCQ paper (or part of one) using their natural degree of caution only. Then they should go through it again being more courageous with their answers (i.e. answering more questions). If the original, natural, degree of caution involved ticking only those questions for which they were absolutely sure of the answers, then almost certainly they will obtain a higher score by guessing some more. My usual advice is to guess at all of those questions that you understand completely, although you are not sure of the correct answer. Guessing at questions that you don't really understand would probably be *too* adventurous.

Another suggestion is to compare, in your first attempt at answering the MCQs, the number of correct answers and the number of false answers. If the ratio of correct:false is of the order of 10:1 (or possibly 5:1) then you will almost certainly improve your score by guessing more. If it is more like 1:1 (or even 2:1) then there is little room for improving your score by guessing more adventurously. I hope that you find these tips helpful.

I am sure that you will find Dr Patel's book a great help in preparing for the MRCPsych Part II.

R. G. PRIEST

PREFACE

This book is based on many years' experience of clinical psychiatry and of guiding trainees through their examinations. It is aimed at doctors preparing for Part II of the MRCPsych examination, and their trainers, though other doctors and medical students may also find it useful in learning about psychiatry and psychiatric examinations. It is my hope that examinees will find it informative and challenging and that its use will allow them to become familiar with both the subject matter and the format of Part II, leading to their safe passage through the examination.

I am sure there is plenty of room for improvement. Constructive criticism, suggestions, new ideas and advice will be warmly welcomed. I have tried to cover as many topics as possible in all sections of the book. Due to limited space, however, it has not been possible to be completely comprehensive. Similarly, I have made every effort to verify the accuracy and appropriateness of the questions and answers that appear in the book, but, as in any text, some inaccuracies and ambiguities may have slipped through. If in doubt, do consult other references as suggested in the Further Reading section.

I would like to thank Dr Hagen Rampes for his contributions to the Basic Science MCQ Papers 1 and 2 and Dr Sagdun Bhandari for his contributions to the Basic Science MCQ Paper 3 and the Clinical Psychiatry Paper 1.

I would also like to thank Professor R. G. Priest for his most helpful advice and his generosity in providing a Foreword.

My sincere thanks are due to the staff of W. B. Saunders for their encouragement, advice and assistance during the preparation of the book.

It would not have been possible to produce this work without my beloved wife and children.

A.G.P.

CONTRIBUTORS

Hagen Rampes
MB BS, MRCPsych
Registrar in Psychiatry
Fairfield Hospital
Hitchin, Hertfordshire
MCQ Basic Science Papers 1 & 2

Sadgun Bhandari
MB BS, MRCPsych
Registrar in Psychiatry
Fairfield Hospital
Hitchin, Hertfordshire
MCQ Basic Science Paper 3
Clinical Psychiatry Paper 1

Ashok G. Patel
MRCPsych, DPM
Consultant Psychiatrist
Fairfield Hospital
Hitchin, Hertfordshire

FORMAT OF THE MRCPSYCH PART II EXAMINATION

Day One

1. One Short Answer Questions paper:
   20 Questions
   Time allowed: 90 minutes

2. One Traditional Essay paper:
   1 out of 6 Questions
   Time allowed: 90 minutes

3. Multiple Choice Questions paper:
   Sciences basic to psychiatry: 50 Questions
   Time allowed: 90 minutes

4. Multiple Choice Questions paper:
   Clinical Psychiatry: 50 Questions
   Time allowed: 90 minutes

Day Two

1. Clinical examination (Long Case):
   Time allowed: 60 minutes to interview the
   patient and 30 minutes with a
   pair of examiners

2. Patient Management Problems/Oral Examination:
   Time allowed: 30 minutes with another pair of
   examiners

THE TRADITIONAL ESSAY PAPER
GUIDELINES

Only *one* out of six questions, which are to be answered in 90 minutes.

Approximately four questions are taken from clinical psychiatry and two questions from sciences basic to psychiatry. Some of the questions may be integrated.

Recent papers have required critical assessment by candidates of important research findings or statements which have appeared in the leading psychiatric and medical journals. Some questions may require critical appraisal of some government policies, discussion papers and other documents, such as *The Health of Nation*.

The purpose of the paper

This is as follows:

  (a) To test candidates' ability to formulate ideas and write in essay form.
  (b) To test candidates' ability to express themselves clearly and without ambiguity.
  (c) To assess candidates' ability to evaluate the evidence critically and produce balanced arguments.
  (d) To test candidates' ability to reproduce what they have learned, with particular reference to literature and research findings.
  (e) Answers should refer to the basic scientific as well as to clinical aspects of each question.

Preparation for the Essay Paper is often a neglected aspect of the membership examination.

Analyse recent examination papers. You may get some idea about topics which are likely to appear in a future examination. Reading textbooks is not enough for this paper. Wide-ranging review of leading journals is an essential aspect of preparation for the examination.

Read all the questions carefully, and then decide which questions you can answer best out of six given questions. Then decide which is the question you can answer best.

Read the chosen question carefully several times. Look for the key words or phrases.

Outline a framework for your answer by 'brain-storming'. It is worth while spending 5 to 10 minutes in this exercise, as you may not have sufficient time to complete another question in the remaining time.

You are expected to cover 4 to 6 pages in your answer, but there is no minimum or maximum number of pages.

You should think of the different angles from which the question might be answered, as such viewpoints may be appreciated as long as the answer is relevant.

Define your terms, definitions, phrases or key words at the outset, as many of them can have a number of meanings.

Tables and diagrams may be used to enhance the clarity of answers.

Each essay should be divided into different sections; for example, introduction, definitions, critical appraisal, discussion, conclusion.

Write legibly, in good English, with due regard to grammar, syntax, spelling and punctuation.

Avoid – repetitions;
  – too much personal and anecdotal experience;
  – a journalistic style;
  – referring to semi-relevant references without showing why you have named them and what their findings were.

Remember that the examiners are looking for a thoughtful, balanced, unprejudiced, comprehensive, open-minded but critical and informed viewpoint based upon relevant evidence and sound clinical knowledge.

Last but not least, remember to leave a few minutes to go through your essay and correct any glaring errors of spelling or syntax.

THE TRADITIONAL ESSAY PAPER
EXAMPLE

Discuss critically the role of bereavement as an aetiological factor in mental disorders.

Answer

Key words – critically;
role;
bereavement;
aetiological;
mental disorders.

The question is in fact more complex than it appears at first glance. Be aware of the key words identified above.

The role of bereavement in the causation of mental disorders has been suspected for a long time; for example, in 1917 Sigmund Freud published his work on mourning and melancholia. Unfortunately, little attention was paid to this topic until the late 1950s.

The essay requires a knowledge of:

– Bereavement causing normal and abnormal grief.
– The role of bereavement as a predisposing and a precipitating factor in the causation of mental disorders.
– Important epidemiological and other studies on this topic.

Introduction

Bereavement is a common occurrence. 'Bereavement' literally means to be deprived of someone by death and refers to the state of mourning.

Grief refers to the subjective feelings that are precipitated by the death of a loved one. The term is used synonymously with 'mourning', although in the strictest sense, 'mourning' refers to the processes by which grief is resolved. It is, in fact, the societal expression of post-bereavement behaviour and practices.

Grief can occur as the result of a variety of losses besides the loss of a loved person. For example, it can result from loss of status, loss of a pet or loss of a national figure. Personal, cultural and incidental factors play an important role in determining the particular form of a grief reaction. Every person and every grief is different.

The expression of grief encompasses a wide range of emotions and behaviours. Grief work is a complex psychological process of withdrawal of attachment and the working through the pain of bereavement.

There are varieties of grief reactions following a bereavement, the commonest being normal grief. The other varieties, like delayed, inhibited or denied grief, refer to the absence of the expression of grief at the time of the loss, when it ordinarily would be expected.

Prolonged or pathological grief is an unusual grief process which goes on beyond the usual period of resolution; namely, a year with intense features.

'Anticipatory grief' is a term which is applied to grief expressed in advance of a loss that is perceived as inevitable, as distinct from grief that occurs at or after the loss. By definition, anticipatory grief ends with the occurrence of anticipated loss, regardless of what reactions follow. Interestingly, unlike the normal grief reaction, which diminishes in intensity with the passage of time, anticipatory grief may increase in intensity as the expected loss becomes more imminent.

The aetiological role in mental disorders

Bereavement, as mentioned earlier, is a common occurrence in our lives. It is, therefore, necessary to examine whether the association between bereavement and mental disorders could be due to chance alone. Its aetiological role, if any, should be considered as a predisposing, precipitating and/or maintaining factor in mental disorders. Aetiology is the bugbear of psychiatry. There are very few mental disorders whose causes are straightforward. Psychiatrists often disagree regarding the cause of a neurotic or a psychotic illness. Despite Freud's insistence on the importance of mourning (Freud, 1917), the reactions to bereavement have received little attention until recent years.

Grief is the only functional psychiatric disorder whose cause is known, whose features are distinctive and whose course is usually predictable. From the currently available knowledge it is not possible to differentiate exactly the role of bereavement as a predisposing or precipitating factor. However, there is some evidence to support its role as an aetiological factor in certain mental disorders.

Apart from grief (which is the link between bereavement and mental disorders), two other factors play an important role in determining the overall reaction to a bereavement. They are stigma and deprivation. Stigma refers to the change in attitude that takes place in society when a person dies. Expressions of sympathy often have a hollow ring and offers of help are often not followed up.

Deprivation refers to the absence of a necessary person or thing, as opposed to the loss of that person or thing. It also implies the absence of those essential 'supplies' that were previously provided by the lost person. A bereaved person reacts to both loss and deprivation. The loss of a husband or wife is one of the most severe forms of psychological stress, one that many of us expect to undergo at some time in our lives. People vary widely in the extent to which they cope with this type of stress (Parkes, 1986).

Compelling evidence suggests that, during grief, the individual is in a vulnerable physical state of biological disequilibrium. Clinical evidence and research findings support the hypothesis that bereavement may be a factor in the development of a wide range of physical and emotional disorders, including fatal illness.

Among the various mental disorders (such as depression, anxiety, panic disorder, hypochondriasis and so on) that can be precipitated by bereavement, the most frequent are likely to comprise atypical forms of grief. These atypical forms of grief differ in intensity and duration from typical (normal) grief (Parkes, 1985).

Bereavement plays an important role in producing depression – a very common single psychiatric diagnosis (Bornstein et al., 1973; Clayton et al., 1972, 1974). People who have experienced depression in the past are more likely to experience depression, rather than normal grief, at the time of a major loss. There is an increased incidence of depressive disorders and suicide attempts in adults who in early childhood experienced the death of a parent. Bowlby (1963) suggested that children who suffer the loss of a parent, particularly the loss of their mother during childhood, may be predisposed to clinging behaviour and excessive grief later in life.

Birtchnell (1975a) found that females who lost a mother before the age of 11 scored highly on 'dependency'. Many became chronic worriers and vulnerable to depression later in life. Birtchnell (1975b) also found that among depressed patients the proportion of women who had lost a father and men who had lost a mother in the preceding five years was about 50 per cent higher than in the general population. The death of a father was also common in alcoholic patients of both sexes. In general, marriage seems to protect people from the traumatic effects of the death of parents.

McMahon and Pugh (1965) found an increased risk of suicide in the four years following widowhood, and was marked among men. Clayton et al. (1974) found that 35 per cent of a sample of bereaved widows over the age of 62 met the criteria of Feighner et al. (1972) for a depressive disorder. About 75 per cent of widows had consulted their general practitioners within six months of bereavement for anxiety, depression, panic and other psychological symptoms (Parkes, 1965; Parkes et al., 1969; Parkes and Brown, 1972).

Psychodynamic aspects of the role of bereavement

Freud (1917) wrote that normal grief (mourning) resulted from the withdrawal of libido from its attachment to the lost person. The self-accusation often seen in depressed patients was really a disguised accusation against someone else for whom he 'felt affection'. He also proposed that depressed patients regress to an earlier stage of development, the oral stage, at which sadistic feelings are powerful. Other psychoanalytic theorists have stressed the role of unconscious and ambivalent factors (such as anger towards the deceased) in grief reactions. The greater the role of these factors, the greater is the likelihood of an abnormal grief reaction. Karl Abraham described the introjection of an ambivalently loved lost object and the subsequent direction of anger towards the introjected object.

Conclusion

There is some evidence of an association between life events and the onset of psychiatric illness (Brown *et al.*, 1973; Brown and Harris, 1978, 1986). Bowlby (1980) has provided convincing evidence of relationships between loss and depression.

Grief may not produce physical pain but it is very unpleasant. It usually disturbs the biological and psychological functions. It is indicated that mental illnesses that follow bereavement often seem to take the form of pathological forms of grieving. Bereavement is also known to precipitate schizophrenia, manic state and various psychosomatic symptoms.

The outcome of bereavement depends on various factors: (a) antecedent: childhood experiences, relationship with the deceased; (b) concurrent: sex, age, premorbid personality; and (c) subsequent: stress, social isolation, emergent life opportunities.

Bereavement is the cause of grief reaction, and it seems to predispose individuals to certain psychiatric disorders while acting as a precipitating factor in others.

References

Birtchnell, J. (1975a) 'The personality characteristics of early-bereaved psychiatric patients', *Social Psychiatry*, 10: 97–103.

Birtchnell, J. (1975b) 'Psychiatric breakdown following recent parent death', *British Journal of Medical Psychology*, 48: 379–90.

Bornstein, P. E., Clayton, P. J., Halikas, J. A., Maurice, W. L. and Robins, E. (1973) 'The depression of widowhood at three months', *British Journal of Psychiatry*, 122: 561–66.

Bowlby, J. (1963) 'Pathological mourning and childhood mourning', *Journal of the American Psychoanalytic Association*, 11: 500.

Bowlby, J. (1980) *Attachment and Loss*, vol. 3, *Loss, Sadness, Depression*, New York: Basic Books.

Brown, G. W., Monck, E. M., Carstairs, G. M. and Wing, J. K. (1962) 'Influence of family life on the cause of schizophrenic illness', *British Journal of Preventive and Social Medicine*, 16: 55–68.

Brown, G. W. and Harris, T. O. (1978) *Social Origins of Depression*, London: Tavistock.

Brown, G. W. and Harris, T. O. (1986) 'Stressor, vulnerability and depression: a question of replication', *Psychological Medicine*, 16: 739–44.

Brown, G. W., Harris, T. O. and Peto, J. (1973) 'Life events and psychiatric disorders: the nature of the causal link', *Psychological Medicine*, 3: 159–76.

Clayton, P. J., Halikas, J. A. and Maurice, W. L. (1972) 'The depression of widowhood', *British Journal of Psychiatry*, 120: 71–8.

Clayton, P. J., Herjanic, M., Murphy, G. E. and Woodruff, R. (1974) 'Mourning and depression: their similarities and differences', *Canadian Psychiatric Association Journal*, 19: 309–12.

Feighner, J. P., Robins, E., Guze, S. B., Woodruff, R. A., Winokur, G. and Munoz, R. (1972) 'Diagnostic criteria for use in psychiatric research', *Archives of General Psychiatry*, 26: 57–63.

Freud, S. (1917) *Mourning and Melancholia*. The Standard Edition of the Complete Psychological Works, vol. 14, pp. 243–560. London: Hogarth Press.

Kinsey, A. C., Pomeroy, W. B. and Martin, C. E. (1948) *Sexual Behaviour in the Human Male*, Philadelphia: Saunders.

Leff, J. P., Knipers, L., Berkowitz, R., Everlein-Vries, R. and Sturgeon, D. A. (1982) 'A controlled trial of social intervention in the families of schizophrenic patients', *British Journal of Psychiatry*, 14: 121–34.

Leff, J. P., Knipers, L., Berkowitz, R., Vaughn, C. and Sturgeon, O. C. (1985) 'Life events, relative expressed emotion and maintenance of neuroleptics in schizophrenic relapse', *Psychological Medicine*, 13: 799–806.

McMahon, B. and Pugh, T. F. (1965) 'Suicide in the widowed', *American Journal of Epidemiology*, 81: 23–31.

Parkes, C. M. (1965) 'Bereavement and mental illness'. Part 1. 'A clinical study of grief of bereaved psychiatric patients', Part 2. 'A classification of bereavement reactions', *British Journal of Medical Psychology*, 38: 1.

Parkes, C. M. (1985) 'Bereavement', *British Journal of Psychiatry*, 146: 11–17.

Parkes, C. M. (1986) *Bereavement: Studies of Grief in Adult Life*, Harmondsworth, England: Penguin Books Ltd.

Parkes, C. M., Benjamin, B. and Fitzgerald, R. G. (1969) 'Broken heart: a statistical study of increased mortality among widowers', *British Medical Journal*, 1: 740–3.

Parkes, C. M. and Brown, R. J. (1972) 'Health after bereavement: a controlled study of young Boston widows and widowers', *Psychosomatic Medicine*, 34: 449–61.

Sturgeon, D. A., Turpin, G., Knipers, L., Berkowitz, R. and Leff, J. P. (1984) 'Psychophysiological responses of schizophrenia patients to high and low expressed emotion relatives: a follow up study', *British Journal of Psychiatry*, 145: 62–9.

Vaughn, C. E. and Leff, J. P. (1976) 'The influence of family and social factors on the cause of psychiatric illness', *British Journal of Psychiatry*, 129: 125–37.

SAQs

THE SAQS PAPER
GUIDELINES

1. This paper consists of 20 questions, which are to be answered in 90 minutes; i.e. 4½ minutes per question.

2. Approximately 10 questions will be drawn from clinical psychiatry and the other 10 from basic sciences. However, some questions may be integrated. Their order of appearance is usually random.

3. *No choice* is given, and therefore all 20 questions must be answered within the allotted time.

4. Unlike in the Multiple Choice Questions paper, there are *no* negative marks in this paper. However, it is not wise to make wild guesses, which may create a negative impression.

5. The questions require short answers; for example, definitions, a list or outline of information required, brief notes or explanations.

6. Ask your colleagues who have taken the examination recently about the content and format of the paper, as the Royal College of Psychiatrists does not publish these papers.

7. Each whole question carries an equal mark.

8. I suggest that, first of all, the candidates should go through the paper quickly and note the questions which they feel they are able to answer easily. Start answering these questions first and then move to others.

9. If possible, do not leave any questions unanswered. It is worthwhile making an educated guess.

10. Try to be factual, brief but comprehensive.

11. The answer to each question may need a slightly different style of presentation.

12. A systematic approach will be useful in answering the questions.

BASIC SCIENCES
QUESTIONS

1. List 10 salient features of frontal lobe syndrome.

2. (a) List the names of nuclei in the hypothalamus.
   (b) Outline their 5 functions.

3. (a) Outline the cerebral pathology of multi-infarct dementia.
   (b) Name 8 characteristic features of multi-infarct dementia.

4. Name the telencephalic, diencephalic, mesencephalic and metencephalic structures of the human brain.

5. (a) What do you understand by the term 'biological markers'?
   (b) Write a brief note on them.

6. (a) What do you understand by the terms: 'down regulation' and 'up regulation' of neuro receptors?
   (b) Write a brief note on the applications of the above terms in understanding the effects of the commonly used psychotropic drugs.

7. (a) Make a list of 5 currently available, non-invasive brain imaging techniques.
   (b) Outline the principles and limitations of any two of these techniques.

8. (a) Define a genetic marker.
   (b) List 4 psychiatric disorders in which genetic markers are implicated.
   (c) List 5 laboratory procedures to locate genetic defect in some of the above disorders.

9. (a) What is meant by the term 'social class'?
   (b) Write a brief note on the relationship between social class and psychiatric disorders.

10. (a) Define the term 'ataxia'.
    (b) Write a brief note on 5 types of ataxia.

11. (a) What do you understand by psychometric tests?
    (b) List 8 tests available for assessment of personality.
    (c) Outline 5 limitations of some of the commonly used tests.

12. (a) What do you understand by the term 'genetic counselling'?
    (b) Discuss briefly its relevance in clinical practice.

13. (a) Define the term 'ethology'.
    (b) Write a short note on its contribution to the understanding of human behaviour.

14. (a) List the names of areas of the brain concerned with the control of normal speech.
    (b) List with brief explanation 5 disturbances of speech which may arise from developmental abnormalities or dysfunction of these areas.

15. (a) What do you understand by the term 'self-esteem'?
    (b) Write a brief note on factors which lead to its development, maintenance and loss in adult life.

16. Write a short note on the importance of non-verbal communication in clinical settings.

17. (a) What do you understand by the term 'perception'?
    (b) Outline 10 disturbances of perception.

18. (a) Define the term 'insight'.
    (b) Write a short note on its importance in psychiatry.

19. (a) Define the term 'personality'.
    (b) Write a brief note on the main determinants of an individual's personality characteristics.

20. (a) Define the term 'biofeedback'.
    (b) Name 4 biofeedback techniques available at present.
    (c) List 5 conditions which may benefit from biofeedback.

BASIC SCIENCES
ANSWERS

1. Dorsolateral prefrontal cortex syndrome.
    - Apathy.
    - Decreased drive.
    - Poor grooming.
    - Psychomotor retardation.
    - Aspontaneity.
    - Decreased attention and concentration.
    - Broca's aphasia (dominant lobe lesions).
    - Indifference.
    - Motor preservation.
    - Pallilalia (repetition of sentences or phrases).
    - Difficulty in changing mental sets.
    - Poor abstract thinking.
    - Motor Jacksonian fits.
    - Urinary incontinence.
    or, alternatively orbitomedial frontal cortex syndrome.
    - Withdrawal.
    - Fearfulness.
    - Lability of mood.
    - Explosiveness.
    - Loss of inhibitions.
    - Occasional violent outbursts.
    - Reduced social and ethical control.
    - Errors of judgement.
    - Irritability.
    - Lack of concern for feelings of other people.

2. (a) Periventricular/supraoptic nuclei:
    - Part of the preoptic nucleus.
    - Suprachiasmatic nucleus.
    - Paraventricular nucleus.
    - Infundibular nucleus.

- Posterior nucleus.
Intermediate zone nuclei:
- Part of the preoptic nucleus.
- Anterior nucleus.
- Dorsomedial nucleus.
- Ventromedial nucleus.
- Premamillary nucleus.
Lateral zone nuclei:
- Part of the preoptic nucleus.
- Supraoptic nucleus.
- Lateral nucleus.
- Tuberomamillary nucleus.
- Lateral tuberal nuclei.
(b) Suprachiasmatic nucleus probably acts as an
endogenous neural pace-maker or biological clock.
To produce hypothalamic releasing factors and release
inhibiting factors for various hormones like
corticotrophin, thyrotrophin, etc.
To influence autonomic nervous system.
To play a role in sexual behaviour.
Satiety centre controls eating.
Hunger centre increases eating.
Thirst centre controls thirst.
Thermo-regulation.
Elaboration of emotions such as aggression, fear,
pleasure and reward.
Secretion of oxytocin and vasopressin.

3. (a) Macroscopic features:
- Multiple cerebral infarcts.
- Local or general atrophy of brain with secondary
ventricular dilatation and cyst formation.
- Arteriosclerotic changes in major arteries.
- Thickened adherent meninges.
- Subdural haemorrhage.
- Perivascular rarefaction, particularly in stratum and
thalamus.
Microscopic features:
- Histological changes of infarction and ischaemia.
- Loss and chromatolysis of nerve cells.

- Irregular patches of demyelination may be seen in white matter.
(b) – Acute onset, peaks in sixties and seventies.
- Step-wise deterioration.
- Focal neurological features, for example, abrupt episodes of hemiparesis, sensory change, dysphasia or visual disturbances.
- Nocturnal confusion.
- Fits.
- Fluctuating cognitive impairment.
- Emotional incontinence.
- Depressed mood, lability of mood.
- Relative preservation of personality.

4.   Telencephalon.
- Cerebral cortex.
- Rhinencephalon.
     Olfactory mucosa.
     Olfactory tracts and bulbs.
     A strip of paleocortex from temporal lobe uncus to medial surface of the frontal lobe.
- Corpus stratum.
     Caudate nucleus.
     Lentiform nucleus.
     Globus pallidus.
- Medullary centre.
Diencephalon.
- Thalamus.
- Subthalamus.
- Hypothalamus.
- Epithalamus.
     Habenular nucleus.
     Pineal gland.
Metencephalon.
- Pons.
- Oral part of the medulla oblongata.
- Cerebellum.
Mesencephalon.
- Tectum, corpora quadrigemina.
- Basis pedunculi.

– Tegmentum.
Red nuclei.
Fibre tracts and grey matter surrounding the
cerebral aqueduct.

5. (a) 'Biological markers' are laboratory tests which are
markers only in the sense of indicating an association
(that may be of a varying degree) between a biological
measure and a given clinical condition.
(b) The association between the marker and the clinical
condition may or may not be aetiologically or
pathophysiologically relevant. These laboratory tests
have clear limitations involving sensitivity and
specificity. The 'biological markers' simply serve as
tools to aid rather than eliminate the decision-making
process. There are a few markers identified; for
example, dexamethasone suppression test for
depression (though it is not specific to depression).
Urinary excretion of 3-methoxy-4-hydroxy
phenylglycol (MHPG) in depressed patients has mean
values very similar to those of bipolar affective
disorder. Ventricular brain ratios (VBRs) are relatively
normal in schizophrenia. The biological marker
approach has yielded some relatively promising
suggestions concerning physiological correlates for
schizoaffective disorder. The electroencephalogram
provides another biological marker approach in
psychiatry.

6. (a) 'Down regulation'.
Drug–receptor interactions may be modified by
receptor sensitivity which is influenced by complex
regulatory and homoeostatic factors. Changes occur
in receptor sensitivity after a prolonged stimulation
by agonist drugs. The receptor cells become
refractory to further stimulation. This is called
'down regulation'. The underlying mechanisms of
this state may involve receptor changes, or the
receptor may be concealed within the cell so that it is
no longer exposed to the ligand.

'Up regulation'.
The receptor cells may become super-sensitive after prolonged receptor blockade. This is called 'up regulation'. It may involve synthesis of new receptors so that an increased number of receptors is exposed on the cell surface to their physiological ligands.

(b) Antipsychotic drugs and dopamine.
Both clinical and adverse effects of antipsychotic drugs result from the blockade of dopaminergic receptors. The Parkinsonian and other adverse effects relate to their blockade of dopaminergic neurotransmission, presumably in the nigrostrital tracts. Tardive dyskinesia has been hypothesized to result from a compensatory development of super-sensitive post-synaptic dopamine receptors following chronic blockade.

Antidepressant drugs and noradrenaline and serotonin.
The acute effects of tricyclic antidepressants is to block re-uptake of noradrenaline and serotonin. The new group of selective serotonin uptake inhibitors are thought to have major effects on serotonergic systems.

Psychotropic drugs and acetyl choline.
Many psychotropic drugs, especially of low potency, block muscarinic receptors, thereby causing side-effects of blurred vision, dry mouth and constipation. Excessive blockade of CNS cholinergic receptors causes confusion and delirium.

7. (a) (i)   X-ray Computerized Tomography scan (CT scan).
   (ii) Magnetic Resonance Imaging (MRI).
   (iii) Magnetic Resonance Spectroscopy.
   (iv) Positron Emission Tomography (PET).
   (v) Single Photon Emission.
   (vi) Single Photon Emission Computerized Tomography (SPECT).
   (vii) Doppler ultrasound and transcranial doppler.
   (viii) Surface laser topography.

(ix) SQUID.

(b) (i) CT Scan:

Principles:

X-ray beams pass through a tissue plane in different directions and the emerging X-rays recorded by scintillation counters are reconstructed by computer into radio density maps.

Greater details can be obtained by higher resolution scanning using thinner slices and introduction of contrast.

Limitations:

– Posterior fossa is not well visualized.
– Some lesions may be isodense.
– It gives an anatomical assessment.

Patients with gross hemiparesis may have a normal scan because the cells involved have not infarcted but have shut down, being in a state of critical perfusion.

(ii) MRI:

Principles:

The patient is placed in a strong static magnetic field which causes the proton spin axes of certain nuclei to align. The precession of the protons is augmented by the administration of radio frequency pulses of the same frequency as that of the precession. At the end of each pulse, energy is emitted and the rate of this decay, the relaxation time and proton density are computed into magnetic resonance image.

Limitations:

– The patient must be free of any metal, so that patients who have had previous surgery cannot be imaged; e.g. patients with steel surgical clips, cardiac pace-makers.

8. (a) It is defined as an identified chromosomal locus for which the genomic position is known.

(b) Schizophrenia – cosegregation of partial trisomy of chromosome 5.

Bipolar affective disorder – a locus on the short arm of chromosome 11.
Huntington's chorea – a locus on the tip of the short arm of chromosome 4.
Alzheimer's disease – a locus on chromosome 21.
Fragile X syndrome – a fragile site on X chromosome.

(c) (i)   Denaturation.
(ii) Gene probes.
(iii) Restriction endonucleases.
(iv) Pulsed field gel electrophoresis.
(v)   Autoradiography.
(vi) Southern blotting.
(vii) Recombinant DNA.
(viii) Linkage analysis.

9. (a) The term 'social class' is used in Western countries to denote an individual's position in the society. Its main determinants include education, financial status, occupation type, geographical areas of residence and leisure activities. In Britain, the assessment of social class is based on the occupation groups as defined by the Office of the Registrar General.

(b) The incidence and prevalence of many psychiatric disorders have been noticed to vary with the social class; e.g. schizophrenia has a greater prevalence in lower social classes, while bipolar affective disorders have a greater representation in higher social classes. There is no convincing evidence to suggest a causal relationship between social class and psychiatric disorders.

There is sufficient evidence to suggest that both treated psychiatric disorders and symptoms of psychological distress are found more frequently in the following:
- lower social classes;
- people without meaningful social ties;
- people who do not have useful social roles;
- people who have suffered significant loss of social ties.

It seems that the relationship between social class and psychiatric disorders is complex but important in certain categories.

10. (a) Ataxia is defined as a dysfunction of motor performance where there is a varying degree of impairment of coordination of separate muscles or groups of muscles in order to accomplish a definite motor act.

(b) (i) Sensory ataxia:
The patient raises his feet very suddenly, often abnormally high, and then jerks them forward, bringing them to the ground again with a stamp, and often heel first.

(ii) Spastic ataxia:
The patient walks on a narrow base, has difficulty in bending his knees and drags his feet along as if they were glued to the floor, as is seen in patients with pyramidal lesions.

(iii) Hemiplegic ataxia:
A spastic gait in which only one leg is affected.

(iv) Cerebellar ataxia:
The patient walks on a broad and irregular base, the feet being planted widely apart. The ataxia is equally severe whether the eyes are open or closed.

(v) Festinant gait:
The patient bends forward and advances with rapid, short, shuffling steps and his arms do not swing. In some cases, if he is suddenly pulled backwards he begins to walk backwards and is unable to stop himself.

(vi) Friedreich's ataxia:
It is the commonest of the spino-cerebellar ataxias and of the hereditary diseases of the nervous system. It usually begins in the first or second decade of life with an unsteady gait. As the condition progresses, the gait becomes broad-based and lurching, action tremor appears in both arms and titubation may develop in the head.

11. (a) Psychometric tests refer to measurements of psychological characteristics, for example, behaviour, intelligence, personality, aptitude. These tests allow recording of observations in numerical form, which makes it easier to understand the results. This facilitates communication between different researchers, and the data can easily be compared and contrasted.

(b) (i) Objective (empirical) tests of personality:
- The Minnesota Multiphasic Personality Inventory (popularly known as MMPI).
- The Meyers-Briggs Inventory.
- The California Psychological Inventory (CPI).
- The Eysenck Personality Questionnaire (EPQ).
- The Hostility and Direction of Hostility Questionnaire (HDHQ).
- Q – sort test.
- Cattell's Sixteen Personality Factor (16PF) Questionnaire.
- Milton Clinical Multiaxial Inventory (MCMI).

(ii) Subjective (projection) tests.
- The Rorschach Inkblot Test.
- The Thematic Apperception Test (TAT).
- The Sentence Completion Test (SCT).
- Draw a Person Test.
- Children's Apperception Test (CAT).
- Word association technique.

(c) Limitations:
- MMPI is not a true personality inventory because the score reflects the relative absence or presence of underlying psychopathology but not the personality dimensions.
- One does not really have a theoretical understanding of the connection between the test reponses and the personality characteristics they identify.
- These tests have been helpful but not completely successful in detecting invalid scales.
- MMPI does not adequately sample some of the traits useful in describing the normal personality.
- MCMI needs further validation research. No information is obtained on the severity of disorders.

– Reliability of the Rorschach Test has been generally poor because the interpretation of responses is too dependent on the clinician's judgement.
– The relationship of TAT scores to overt behaviour is complex. The patient's preoccupations are not necessarily acted on.

12. (a) Genetic counselling provides the patients and their families with direct medical knowledge in the field of genetics. It is indicated when there is even the remotest possibility of a genetically based disorder in the family.
   (b) Genetic counselling requires the clinician to be aware of a patient's level of maturity, individual conflicts, defence mechanisms and ego strengths and weaknesses. Its goals include:
      (i)   a realistic and appropriate appreciation of the patient's or spouse's family history;
      (ii)   the communication of current knowledge of a morbid risk;
      (iii) a way to cope with risk related to anxiety and narcissistic injury;
      (iv)   a plan for the appropriate response to high risk;
      (v)   communication of knowledge of relative contributions of environmental factors to aetiology;
      (vi)   the communication of knowledge of the mechanism of inheritance.
   From family studies, it is quite clear that most family members of a Huntington's chorea patient would prefer to have known the diagnosis earlier and to have an opportunity for genetic counselling.

13. (a) Ethology is the study of the behaviour of animals in their natural environments, and the origins of such behaviour.
   (b) It is particularly concerned with the process of development in young animals, of a positive bond between members of the same species, courtship, sexual behaviour and care of the young.
      – The findings of animal studies can shed light on the

understanding of human behaviour; e.g. the bonding and attachment behaviour during the first year of life closely approximate to imprinting behaviour.
- Human beings continue to be attached to their parents regardless of whether their early attachments were optimal. The attachments continue to occur at various stages in life to different persons such as teachers, relatives and older siblings.
- An adult attachment bond provides a sense of security, a sense of being needed and a sense of being able to give. The absence of the attachment figure makes the person feel lonely or anxious.
- The severing of attachments can be traumatic.
- The knowledge of aggression in animals can be applied to human beings.
- Human beings exhibit displacement; for example, it is seen in birds when under stress.
- The common personality disorders bear a strong resemblance to the behaviour of Harlow's Monkeys.
- Psychotropic drug research is dependent on strategies for modifying animal behaviour.

14. (a) The parts of brain concerned with speech are multiple and extensive, and are necessarily diffused over a considerable area.
    - Wernicke's area (first temporal convolution).
    - Broca's area (posterior part of the frontal lobe).
    - Arcuate fasciculus.
    - Thalamus.
    - Corpus striatum.
  (b) (i) Nominal aphasia:
        - An inability to speak words. The principal difficulty lies in evoking names at will. This may vary from total inability to name any object on confrontation to a mild disorder.
     (ii) Pure word deafness:
        - An inability to comprehend spoken speech. The patient can read and comprehend written material.

(iii) Pure word-blindness:
   – An inability to read. The patient can speak
     normally and has no difficulty with
     comprehension of spoken words.
(iv) Broca's dysphasia:
   – The defect is on the effect side of speech,
     concerning with the mechanism by which
     words are chosen, articulated and sentences
     constructed. Speech is characteristically sparse,
     slow and hesitant, with marked disturbances of
     rhythm, inflexion and articulations.
(v) Acalculia:
   – An inability to comprehend symbols; e.g.
     mathematical or musical symbols.
(vi) Apraxia:
   – An inability to make use of objects, though the
     patient can recognize their use.
(vii) Jargon aphasia:
   – Speech is produced freely, volubly and clearly
     but with such semantic jumble and misuse of
     words that meaning cannot be discerned.

15. (a) The term 'self-esteem' is quite often loosely used in
       clinical practice. It means the sense of contentment and
       self-acceptance which stems from a person's appraisal
       of various issues such as his or her own worth,
       significance, competence, attractiveness, confidence
       and ability to satisfy his or her aspirations.
   (b) Self-esteem is a part of an individual's personality.
       According to psychoanalytic theory, it depends not
       only on experiences at the oral stage but also on failure
       at later stages of development.
         It is continuously at risk in human beings, especially
       elderly persons when they lose external sources of
       support. It is maintained and promoted by several
       factors; for example:
       (i) by economic security;
       (ii) by supportive persons who protect them against
           isolation and allow the need for dependency to be
           gratified;

    (iii) by psychological and/or mental health, which
          facilitates mature coping and defence mechanisms;
    (iv) by physical health, which enables the person to
          pursue productive activities.

Loss of self-esteem occurs in various psychiatric disorders; e.g. depression and schizophrenia. When the factors which help to maintain it are affected adversely, it is very likely to be diminished or lost.

16.   By 'non-verbal communication' are denoted all those human responses which are not described as overtly manifested words (either spoken or written).

- In addition to verbal communication, non-verbal communication is an important aspect of the therapeutic relationship. It is more important in the absence of verbal communication in a variety of clinical situations; for example, silent pauses during psychoanalysis, mutism and stupor.
- Evidence of autonomic activity like sweating or flushing may signal that the topic under discussion is emotionally significant. If a patient says that he has non-visible autonomic responses such as palpitations, abdominal pain or headache during the interview, he should be asked to report when they occur.
- Sometimes the patient is unaware of the aspects of his communicative behaviour that upset others. In this connection, a useful manoeuvre is to call the patient's attention to the discrepancies between his verbal and non-verbal communications.
- Video-tape play-back, by sharply confronting patients with the way they present themselves to others, can enhance the outcome of the therapy.
- Non-verbal communication is a part of a collection of interactive behaviours which make up the interchange in a group. Its functions, therefore, have to do with keeping the interaction running smoothly as well as with expressing the feelings, attitudes and personalities of the members in a group.

17. (a) Perception is concerned with the sensation and interpretation of our environment. It therefore comprises the mechanisms and processes that provide a useful representation of the outside world in our brains. It is thus a process of becoming aware of what is being presented through the sensory organs such as ears, eyes, nose and skin.

(b) (i) Hallucinations:
- Hypnagogic hallucination.
- Hypnopompic hallucination.
- Auditory hallucination.
- Visual hallucination.
- Olfactory hallucination.
- Gustatory hallucination.
- Tactile hallucination.
- Somatic hallucination.
- Lilliputian hallucination.
- Synaesthesia.
- Trailing phenomenon.

(ii) Illusions.

(iii) Disturbance associated with organic mental disorder:
- Anosognosia.
- Autotopagnosia.
- Visual agnosia.
- Astereognosia.
- Prosopagnosia.

(iv) Disturbances associated with conversion and dissociative phenomena:
- Macropsia.
- Micropsia.
- Depersonalization.
- Fugue.
- Multiple personality.

18. (a) Insight is defined as the patient's degree of awareness of his or her own mental condition and the need for receiving appropriate treatment.

(b) The accuracy of diagnosis and success of the treatment depend to a large extent on the patient's cooperation with the doctor. While it is true that neurotic patients usually retain insight and psychotic patients lose it, this is not invariable.

When assessing insight, it is important to keep in mind the complexity of the concept. Questions should be tailored to elicit not just the presence or absence of insight but also the level of insight. Intellectual insight is said to be present when patients admit that they are ill and acknowledge that their failure to adapt is, in part, due to their own irrational feelings.

True emotional insight is said to be present when patients' awareness of their own motives and deep feelings lead to change in their personality or behaviour pattern. If the patient is unwilling to cooperate with the clinicians and is considered to be a danger to self and/or others, it may lead to serious consequences, such as, for example, compulsory admission and treatment in a hospital. The level of insight may affect the therapeutic relationship between the doctor and the patient.

19. (a) Personality is defined as the totality of emotional and behavioural traits that characterize a person in day-to-day living under ordinary conditions. It is relatively stable and predictable.

(b) (i) Genetic factors inherited from parents; e.g. temperaments:
There is evidence that temperament is an early building block for later personality traits. It appears to be determined in part by genetic factors, and is inherited from the parents, in spite of wide differences between children of the same family.

(ii) Environmental factors:
Attachment is an infant's tendency to seek closeness to care givers and to feel more secure in their presence.

(iii) Parental child-rearing practices:
After the first year of a child's life, child rearing becomes more complicated as parents take on the tasks of discipline, control and character building.

(iv) Personality–environmental interactions.

(v) Cultural influences:
Different cultures have differing values in the independence and self-assertiveness of children. Individuals who do not conform to the cultural norms are likely to be pressured to change.
In shaping personality, genetic and environmental influences do not act independently of each other but are intertwined from the moment of birth.

(vi) Libido theory:
The theory stresses libido as energy. The child is initially motivated by pleasure received from certain kinds of bodily stimulation and reacts positively to persons from whom such stimuli are received. It also stresses the crucial relationship between child and mother.

20. (a) Biofeedback is an application of operant conditioning in which human subjects are given feedback on the functioning of their autonomic nervous system – for example, blood pressure or motor function – and they can be trained to exert some control over it.

(b) (i) An electromyogram (EMG) measures the electrical potentials of muscle fibres.

(ii) An electroencephalogram (EEG) measures alpha waves that occur in relaxed states.

(iii) Galvanic Skin Response (GSR) shows decreased skin conductivity during a relaxed state.

(iv) Thermistor measures skin temperature, which drops during tension because of peripheral vasoconstriction.

(c) – Migraine.
   – Hypertension.
   – Tension headaches.

- Cardiac arrhythmias.
- Epilepsy.
- Bronchial asthma.
- Myofascial pain.
- Insomnia.
- Hyperactivity in children.

CLINICAL PSYCHIATRY
QUESTIONS

1. (a) List 4 psychiatric defences used in the courts of law in the United Kingdom.
   (b) Describe briefly 2 of these defences.

2. (a) Define the terms 'actus reus' and 'mens rea'.
   (b) Give examples of crimes for which 'specific intent' is required and for which it is not required.

3. Outline 4 indications and 5 contra-indications of group psychotherapy.

4. Outline the main points of assessment of a child who is suspected to have sustained non-accidental injuries.

5. (a) Who coined the term 'schizo-affective disorder'?
   (b) Name 3 features used in the operational definition (DSMIIIR) of this disorder.
   (c) Name 2 biochemical abnormalities which are thought to occur in this disorder.

6. (a) Define the term 'expressed emotion'.
   (b) What is its significance in clinical practice?
   (c) What measures will you take to minimize the untoward effects of high expressed emotion?

7. Discuss briefly the implications of a diagnosis of bulimia nervosa on the patient as well as her family.

8. (a) What do you understand by the term 'punch-drunk syndrome'?
   (b) Give 4 characteristic features of the above condition.
   (c) How will you differentiate it both clinically and pathologically from Alzheimer's disease?

9. Outline how you will assess dangerousness in a mentally disordered patient.

10. (a) Define the term 'phobia'.
    (b) Outline the classification of phobic disorders according to the ICD10 system.
    (c) List 8 salient features of a panic attack.

11. (a) Define the term 'informed consent'.
    (b) List its 5 characteristic features.
    (c) Write a brief note on factors which indicate whether or not the patient is capable of giving informed consent.

12. (a) List 5 common factors in psychotherapies.
    (b) Outline the potential difficulties in psychotherapy research.
    (c) Write a brief note on outcome measures of psychotherapies.

13. (a) What do you understand by the term 'therapeutic community'?
    (b) Outline its underlying principles.

14. Write a short note on 3 types of involuntary movement disorders caused by psychotropic drugs.

15. (a) What do you understand by the term 'cognitive therapy'?
    (b) List 3 goals of cognitive therapy.
    (c) Outline 6 techniques of cognitive therapy.

16. (a) What do you understand by the term 'elective mutism'?
    (b) List its 5 differential diagnoses.
    (c) Outline its treatment plan.

17. (a) What are the characteristic features of post-traumatic stress disorder?
    (b) What differential diagnoses would you consider in such a case of a 50-year-old married woman?

18. List factors considered important in the discharge plan of a compulsorily detained restricted patient.

19. Write brief notes on the information you would give to a patient who was prescribed a long-acting depot neuroleptic drug for the first time.

20. Describe briefly the desirable characteristics of a rating scale.

CLINICAL PSYCHIATRY
ANSWERS

1. (a) (i) Unfit to plead.
   (ii) Not guilty by reasons of insanity ('special verdict').
   (iii) Diminished responsibility.
   (iv) Incapacity to form an intent because of automatism.
   (b) (i) Unfit to plead.
       - Under English law, every defendant must be fit to defend himself or herself against alleged charges.
       - The issue can be raised by the defence, prosecution or a judge, but it can only be decided by a jury.
       - Criteria to assess unfitness to plead – any one or more of the following:
         A) inability to understand the nature of the charge;
         B) inability to understand the significance of his plea;
         C) inability to instruct counsel;
         D) inability to challenge jurors;
         E) inability to examine a witness;
         F) inability to follow the progress of the trial.
         A person may be suffering from a severe mental disorder but may still be fit to stand trial. If the defendant is unfit to plead, an order is made to admit him or her to a hospital specified by the Home Secretary until he or she is fit to stand trial.
   (ii) Not guilty by reason of insanity ('special verdict').
       - This concept is embodied in the McNaghton Rules, which have no statutory basis but are

accepted by the courts as having the status of law.

- Defined as 'To establish a defence on the ground of insanity, it must be clearly proved that at the time of committing the act, the party accused was labouring under such a defect of reason, from disease of the mind, as not to know the nature and the quality of the act he was doing, or if he did know it, that he did not know what he was doing was wrong'.

If the defence is successful, the court must order the defendant's admission to a hospital decided by the Home Secretary. It has been used less in murder cases since the abolition of the death penalty in the United Kingdom.

2. (a) Actus reus: The prosecution must prove that the defendant has carried out an unlawful act. Mens rea: The prosecution must prove that the defendant was in a guilty state of mind at the time of the alleged offence. It is often loosely referred to as 'a guilty mind'.
   (b) Crimes for which 'specific intent' is required:
   - murder,
   - arson,
   - rape,
   - assault with intent to cause grievous bodily harm.
   Crimes for which 'specific intent' is not required:
   - crimes committed by children under the age of 10,
   - traffic offences,
   - manslaughter,
   - indecent assault,
   - assault occasioning actual bodily harm.

3. *Indications of group psychotherapy:*
   In addition to the conventional diagnostic categories in selection, a useful approach is to consider the patient's presenting complaints and to add any pertinent dynamic problems that are free from undue inference or speculation.

(a) Self-concept – lack of clear identity, low self-esteem, lack of purpose and direction.
(b) Symptomatic – anxiety, depression, somatization, ineffective coping with stress.
(c) Emotional – unawareness of feeling, inability to express feelings like love or anger, poor control over emotions.
(d) Interpersonal functioning – inability to achieve intimacy, inability to maintain a heterosexual relationship.

Contra-indications of group psychotherapy:
The patients who do poorly include:
(a) the severe depressive,
(b) the acute schizophrenic,
(c) the paranoid personality,
(d) the extreme schizoid,
(e) the sociopath,
(f) the hypochondriacal type,
(g) the narcissist,
(h) the drug-dependent patient and the alcoholic.

4. Assessment of a child with suspected non-accidental injuries:
   - Suspicion should be aroused by the pattern of physical injuries, previous history of suspicious injury, unconvincing explanations, delay in seeking medical help and incongruous parental reactions.
   - History from the child, parents and other reliable sources.
   - Clinical features of the child and relevant case history:
     - premature birth,
     - early separation,
     - need for special care in baby unit,
     - congenital malformation,
     - chronic illness,
     - difficult temperament,
     - fearful responses to parents,
     - undue anxiety or unhappiness,
     - low self-esteem.

- Parental factors associated with child abuse:
  - youth,
  - social isolation,
  - marital disharmony/relationship problems with the partner,
  - criminal record,
  - antisocial personality, especially of the father,
  - family violence,
  - poor socioeconomic status.
- Admission to hospital for further assessment:
  - through physical examination,
  - photographs of injuries,
  - skeletal X-rays,
  - CT scan if subdural haemorrhage is suspected.

5. (a) Jacob Kasanin (1933) coined the term 'Schizo-affective disorder'.

   (b) (i) A disturbance during which there is either a major depressive or a manic syndrome concurrent with characteristic symptoms of schizophrenia.

   (ii) During an episode of the disturbance, there have been delusions or hallucinations for at least 2 weeks but no prominent mood symptoms.

   (iii) Diagnosis of schizophrenia has been ruled out.

   (iv) It cannot be established that an organic factor initiated and maintained the disturbance.

   (c) (i) There is a hyperactivity of the dopaminergic system.

   (ii) There is a possibility of increased noradrenergic activity.

   (iii) There is a possibility of a reduced gamma amino butyric acid activity.

6. (a) Expressed emotion is characterized by critical comments, hostile feelings and intrusiveness on the part of families of schizophrenic patients.

   (b) Brown et al. (1962) found that relapse rates of schizophrenia were greater in families where relatives showed high expressed emotion. In such families, the risk of relapse was greater if the patients were in contact with their close relatives for more than 35 hours a week.

A psychophysiological investigation (Sturgeon *et al.*, 1984) reported an association between expressed emotion in a close relative and the level of autonomic arousal recorded in the patient, suggesting that such arousal may be a mediating variable.

Vaughn and Leff (1976) suggested an association between expressed emotion in relatives and the patient's response to antipsychotic drugs.

Leff *et al.* (1982, 1985a,b) strongly suggest that high expressed emotion has a causal role in relapse of schizophrenic illness.

(c) Discharge of schizophrenic patients to neutral accommodation, such as a staffed/unstaffed hostel or group home.

Daytime therapeutic activities.

Regular maintenance on neuroleptic drugs.

Family therapy, education, expressed emotion reduction programme, social network maintenance.

7. *Patient:*
   (a) Psychological:
   Depressive symptoms which may require antidepressant drugs are common.
   (b) Physical:
   Repeated vomiting may lead to electrolyte imbalance, dehydration, loss of potassium, resulting in weakness, cardiac arrhythmia.
   Renal damage.
   Urinary infections.
   Tetany and epileptic fits may occur.
   (c) Treatment plan will need to be worked out.
   Family:
   Psychological: stress, guilt, tensions.
   Aetiological factors:
   – families are less close, more conflictual than the families of anorexic girls,
   – parents described as neglectful and rejecting,
   – treatment aspects – involvement of the family may be necessary.

8. (a) It is a controversial term applied to 'punch-drunkenness' seen in retired boxers. Some of the supporters of boxing seek to explain it on the grounds of coincidentally occurring neurological disease or alcoholism rather than the boxing career. The syndrome's clinical features appear to follow repeated mild head injuries, each in itself leading to no more than brief concussion.

(b) Neurological features:
All grades of cerebellar, pyramidal and extra-pyramidal disorders of varying degree:
   - dysarthria,
   - facial immobility,
   - poverty and slowness of movement,
   - ataxia,
   - tremor of hands and head,
   - spasticity of limbs.
Psychiatric features:
   - intellectual and personality deterioration; e.g. irritability, progressive apathy, rage reactions,
   - chronic amnesic state,
   - morbid jealousy,
   - progressive dementia.

(c) It differs from Alzheimer's disease as follows:
Clinical features:
   - patients have a history of boxing, persistent headache, dizziness, fatigue and inability to concentrate,
   - concomitant coexistence of dysarthria, ataxia, Parkinsonism and pyramidal disorders.
Macroscopic picture of the brain:
   - cerebral atrophy,
   - cerebellar atrophy,
   - perforation of the septum pellucidum ('cavum septum pellucidum').
Microscopic picture of the brain:
   - extensive loss of neurones in cerebral cortex and presence of neurofibrillary tangles without neuritic plaques,
   - cerebral degeneration is concentrated near the septal region.

9. Assessment of dangerousness:
    - Difficult but vital.
    - No fixed rules for assessing dangerousness.
    - The following guidelines apply to both offenders as well as non-offenders:
    (a) Do not rely entirely on your own evaluation of dangerousness but discuss the problem with other significant colleagues and relatives.
    (b) History:
        - previous episodes of violence,
        - repeated impulsive behaviour,
        - any consistent pattern of behaviour,
        - difficulty in coping with stress,
        - previous unwillingness to delay gratification,
        - sadistic or paranoid personality traits.
    (c) Offence:
        - characteristics of the current offence,
        - bizarre violence,
        - continuing denial of the offence,
        - lack of remorse or guilt.
    (d) Mental state examination:
        - pathological jealousy,
        - paranoid beliefs/delusions and a wish to harm other people,
        - lack of self-control,
        - threat to repeat violence,
        - insight.
    (e) Circumstances:
        - provocation or precipitant likely to occur,
        - alcohol or drug abuse,
        - lack of social support,
        - social difficulties.

10. (a) Phobia is defined as an irrational fear which is:
        (i)   out of proportion to the demand of the situation,
        (ii) cannot be explained or reasoned away,
        (iii) beyond voluntary control, and which
        (iv) leads to an avoidance of the feared object or situation.

(b) (i) simple phobia,
    (ii) social phobia,
    (iii) agoraphobia.

(c) Salient features of a panic attack:
    (i) shortness of breath and smothering sensations,
    (ii) choking,
    (iii) palpitations,
    (iv) chest discomfort or pain,
    (v) sweating,
    (vi) dizziness or faintness,
    (vii) nausea or abdominal distress,
    (viii) trembling,
    (ix) fear of dying,
    (x) fear of going crazy.

11. (a) Informed consent is the cornerstone of autonomy theory. Adult patients are assumed to have the right to consent or refuse consent to treatment. The document of informed consent serves only as a record of completion of a process which should include enough uncoerced time and information to make an informed choice about investigations or treatment.

(b) (i) Language understandable to the layman.
    (ii) Description of the procedures to be followed.
    (iii) Description of any reasonable foreseeable risks and discomforts to the patient.
    (iv) Description of any benefits to the patient or others.
    (v) Disclosure of appropriate alternative procedures.
    (vi) Statement of confidentiality.
    (vii) Voluntary participation.
    (viii) Consent can be withdrawn at any time without prejudice.

(c) The following can influence a patient's ability to give an informed consent:
    (i) mental handicap/learning difficulties,
    (ii) young age,
    (iii) severe psychotic illness,
    (iv) patient detained compulsorily under Mental Health Act.

12. (a) Common factors in psychotherapies:
    - an interpersonal relationship of warmth and trust,
    - reassurance and support,
    - desensitization,
    - reinforcement of adaptive responses,
    - understanding or insight.
    (b) - definition of psychotherapy treatments,
    - controls in psychotherapy,
    - power and sample size,
    - measurement of outcome,
    - generalization of results.
    (c) Outcome measures may look at:
    - psychodynamic change,
    - symptom relief,
    - social adaptation, or
    - a combination of the above.
    The measures chosen to look at outcome in psychotherapy must then be capable of accurately measuring the specific outcome variables being considered. The timing of studies is important. The outcome research should attempt to address the question of whether or not benefits are maintained. The measures must be clearly definable and measurable. The most common outcome designs include:
    (i) no treatment group,
    (ii) placebo control,
    (iii) comparative treatment group.

13. (a) It is an in-patient psychotherapeutic unit for the treatment of antisocial personalities. In such a unit, the patients live and work together and meet several times a day for group discussions in which each person's behaviour and feelings are examined by other members of the group. It is hoped that, by repeating this process over a period of time, the patients will gradually learn to control their antisocial behaviour and feelings. This may eventually lead to better ways of coping with their life.

(b) Rapoport described 4 basic principles:
(i) Democratization – abolition of hierarchy.
(ii) Permissiveness – tolerance of disturbed behaviour.
(iii) Reality confrontation – regular feedback to the individuals of the results of their behaviour.
(iv) Communalism – equal shares for all.

14. Psychotropic drugs include antipsychotics, antidepressants, hypnotics, anxiolytics, lithium carbonate and carbamazepine. Three types of involuntary movement disorders are described below:
(a) Acute dystonia:
Occurs soon after the treatment with antipsychotics begins, especially in young men.
It is characterized by:
– torticollis,
– tongue protrusion,
– grimacing,
– opisthotonus.
It can easily be mistaken for histrionic behaviour.
(b) Akathisia:
Usually occurs within the first 2 weeks of starting treatment with antipsychotic drugs, but may begin only after several months.
It is an unpleasant feeling of physical restlessness and a need to move, leading to an inability to keep still.
When it occurs early, it disappears if the dose is reduced overall; it is not reliably controlled by anti-Parkinsonian drugs.
(c) Parkinsonian syndrome:
It appears after a few weeks of starting the treatment with antipsychotic drugs. It is characterized by:
– akinesia,
– expressionless face ('mask-like face'),
– lack of associated swinging movements of arms,
– rigidity,
– coarse tremors,
– stooped posture,
– festinant gait.

The symptoms can be controlled by reduction in dosage of antipsychotic drugs and/or by anti-Parkinsonian drugs.

(d) Tardive dyskinesia:

It is more common in women and the elderly. The exact cause of the syndrome is unknown but it could be supersensitivity to dopamine resulting from prolonged dopaminergic blockade. No universally effective treatment is available.

It is characterized by:
- chewing and sucking movements,
- grimacing,
- choreoathetoid movements,
- akathisia.

15. (a) A term applied to psychological treatments intended to change maladaptive ways of thinking and thereby bring about improvement in psychiatric disorders. It is orientated towards current problems and their solution.

(b) Goals:
- To alleviate depression or other problems and to prevent its recurrence by helping the patient.
- To identify and test negative cognitions.
- To develop alternative and more flexible schemes.
- To rehearse both new cognitive and new behavioural responses.
- To change the way the patient thinks and to alleviate the distressing symptoms.

(c) Techniques of cognitive therapy:
- Eliciting automatic thoughts.
- Testing automatic thoughts.
- Identifying maladaptive underlying assumptions.

Cognitive behavioural techniques:
- Scheduling activities.
- Mastery and pleasure.
- Graded task assignments.
- Cognitive rehearsal.
- Self-reliance training.
- Role playing.
- Diversion techniques.

16. (a) Elective mutism is characterized by a persistent refusal to talk about one or more major social situations, including at school, despite the ability to comprehend spoken language and to speak. It is a psychologically determined inhibition or refusal to speak. The speech is limited only to certain family members. More girls than boys are affected.

(b) Differential diagnosis:
   - Mental retardation.
   - Pervasive developmental disorders.
   - Developmental expressive language disorder.
   - A psychotic disorder.
   - Hearing impairment.

(c) Multimodal approach consisting of:
   - Individual, behavioural and family interventions.
   For pre-school child:
   - Psychotherapy or counselling of parents.
   - A therapeutic nursery for the child.
   For school-age child:
   - Individual psychotherapy.
   - Behavioural psychotherapy.
   - When a child's independence is being thwarted, marital counselling or psychotherapy for parents is of paramount importance.

17. (a) – The person has experienced a traumatic event that is outside the usual range of human experience and that would be markedly distressing to almost anyone.
   - The traumatic event is persistently re-experienced in many ways; e.g.
      - recurrent and intrusive distressing recollections of the event,
      - recurrent distressing dreams of the event.
   - Persistent avoidance of the stimuli and place of the incident.
   - Persistent symptoms of increased arousal; e.g.
      - difficulty in falling or staying asleep,
      - irritability or outbursts of anger,
      - difficulty with concentration,

     – hyper-vigilance,
     – exaggerated startle response.
   – Duration of symptoms of at least one month.
  (b) Differential diagnosis:
     (i)   Head injury.
     (ii)   Alcohol dependence.
     (iii) Drug dependence.
     (iv) Factitious disorder.
     (v)   Malingering.
     (vi) Borderline personality disorder.
     (vii) Adjustment reaction.
     (viii) Depression.
     (ix) Panic disorder.
     (x)   Generalized anxiety disorder.

18.   – Read carefully the judgement delivered by the Mental Health Review Tribunal.
      – Accommodation required, whether supervised or unsupervised.
      – Medical supervision by the responsible medical officer.
      – Pharmacological treatment.
      – Daytime activities.
      – Social worker involvement.
      – Community psychiatric nurse involvement.
      – Re-admission facilities.
      – Regular reports to the Home Secretary.
      – Involvement of the carers.
      – Approval of the discharge plan by the Tribunal.

19.   – Information about the clinical diagnosis.
      – Rationale for long-term treatment.
      – Consequences of inadequate treatment; e.g. repeated breakdowns, re-admissions.
      – How long the treatment is likely to last.
      – Description of the prescribed medication.
      – Dosage and frequency.
      – Who will administer the drug.
      – Side-effects profile.

- Early-warning signs of relapse of the condition.
- Alternatives to depot injections.

20. – A rating scale records the characteristic of the subjects in numerical form so that it can be assessed quantitatively.
- It should be able to offer screening and diagnosis.
- It should be sensitive to change in the patient's condition.
- It should be valid; i.e. it should measure what it is supposed to measure.
- It should be reliable; i.e. repeatable.
- It should have a satisfactory level of sensitivity.
- It should have a satisfactory level of specificity.
- It should be user-friendly.

References

Brown, G. W., Monck, E. M., Carstairs, G. M. and Wing, J. K. (1962) 'Influence of family life on the cause of schizophrenic illness', *British Journal of Preventive and Social Medicine*, 16: 55–68.

Kasanin, J. (1933) 'The acute schizo-affective psychoses', *American Journal of Psychiatry*, 13: 97–126.

Leff, J. P., Knipers, L., Berkowitz, R., Everlein-Vries, R. and Sturgeon, D. A. (1982) 'A controlled trial of social intervention in the families of schizophrenic patients', *British Journal of Psychiatry*, 14: 121–34.

Leff, J. P., Knipers, L., Berkowitz, R. and Sturgeon, D. (1985a) 'A controlled trial of intervention in the families of schizophrenic patients: two year follow up', *British Journal of Psychiatry*, 146: 594–600.

Leff, J. P., Knipers, L., Berkowitz, R., Vaughn, C. E. and Sturgeon, D. (1985b) 'Life events, relative expressed emotion and maintenance of neuroleptics in schizophrenic relapse', *Psychological Medicine*, 13: 799–806.

Sturgeon, D., Turpin, G., Knipers, L., Berkowitz, R. and Leff, J. (1984) 'Psychophysiological responses of schizophrenia patients to high and low expressed emotion relatives: a follow up study', *British Journal of Psychiatry*, 145: 62–69.

Vaughn, C. E. and Leff, J. P. (1976) 'The influence of family and social factors on the cause of psychiatric illness', *British Journal of Psychiatry*, 129: 125–37.

MCQs

THE MCQS PAPERS
GUIDELINES

Each question consists of a stem followed by five suggested answers. The candidates are asked to indicate whether each answer is true or false or to state 'Don't know'. There is no restriction on the number of true or false answers in any individual question. However, it is believed that approximately 50 per cent of answers are true and the rest are false.

Negative marking

The answers correctly identified as true or false receive a mark of +1. Those marked as 'Don't know' receive a zero mark, while incorrectly identified answers (that is, true as false and false as true answers) receive a penalty mark of −1.

Guesswork is therefore not rewarding and may be damaging. However, I suggest that some degree of gamble may be required to achieve a pass mark.

Develop a clear understanding of various terms used in these questions as well as the format and style of the question.

All the answers are independent of one another; in other words, one cannot derive a clue about an answer from another.

The first impression is often the best, so beware of making changes unless they are based on insight.

Read each paper carefully and answer the questions under strict examination conditions. This will help you to identify your strengths and weaknesses. Having done this, refer to the given answers and explanations.

If you understand the stem of the question thoroughly, it is worthwhile making a guess, but if you are unsure it is advisable not to guess.

Practise according to these principles in order to assess your knowledge as follows:

(a) Don't know but would guess.
(b) Don't know and would not guess.

Two methods to use to answer the MCQ papers

It is a matter of choice for each examinee to use one of these methods, but I personally recommend the first method in the examination.

1. Mark all the answers as 'T' for true, 'F' for false or 'D' for 'Don't know' on the question paper. Then carefully transfer all the answers onto the answer sheet provided. Make sure that all the answers are marked in the correct boxes.

   I believe that it is much easier to transfer the answers to the answer sheet than to answer the questions and mark the answer sheet when there is a shortage of time. This technique may also allow some spare time to revisit outstanding queries in the paper.

2. Answer the questions as you go; read and mark them on the answer sheet immediately. Repeat the process until you reach the last question. It may be that you will find some questions difficult to answer correctly; if so, leave them and proceed to the next question. Revisit the unanswered questions.

There is no minimum or maximum number of answers to the questions for a pass mark. I would advise you to answer confidently as many questions as you can.

EXPLANATION OF TERMS USED IN MCQS

There is a consensus that the following terms have the following implied meanings:

1. **Occurs:**
   Makes no statement about frequency (i.e. a recognized occurrence).

2. **Recognized:**
   Has been reported as a feature or association.

3. **Characteristic or typical:**
   Features that occur so often as to be of some diagnostic significance and whose absence might lead to some doubt being cast on diagnosis.

4. **Essential/diagnostic feature:**
   Must occur to make a diagnosis.

5. **Specific or pathognomic:**
   Features that occur in the named disease and no other.

6. **Can be or may be:**
   It is recognized (i.e. reported) as occurring.

7. **Commonly, frequently, is likely or often:**
   Imply a rate of occurrence greater than 50%.

8. **Always or never:**
   Suggest that there are no recognized exceptions.

9. **Particularly associated:**
   The association is significant in samples with sufficient numbers.

10. **Exclusively:**
    Features that occur in the named condition and no others.

11. **Invariably:**
    Implies the occurrence of a feature without a shadow of doubt.

12. **Only:**
    Singles out a feature or a condition.

13. **Include:**
    Like 'occurs', makes no mention of frequency.

14. **Majority:**
    Means 50% or more.

15. **Implicit:**
    Implied though not plainly expressed, virtually contained.

16. **Explicit:**
    Expressly stated, leaving nothing merely implied, stated in detail.

17. **Usually:**
    60% or more.

BASIC SCIENCES
PAPER 1

1. *The following statements about cognitive dissonance are correct:*
   (a) It is a concept originally developed by social psychologists.
   (b) It is usually found in patients suffering from social phobia.
   (c) It is normally found in patients suffering from bipolar affective disorder.
   (d) It makes for low self-esteem.
   (e) It is a cause of internal comfort in human beings.

2. *According to the psychoanalytic theory of dreams, the following mental mechanisms are involved:*
   (a) Projective identification.
   (b) Projection.
   (c) Secondary revision.
   (d) Desymbolization.
   (e) Dissociation.

3. *Most psychoanalysts would agree that anal eroticism leads to:*
   (a) Sodomy.
   (b) Homosexuality.
   (c) Miserliness.
   (d) Bestiality.
   (e) Obsessional traits.

4. *The following statements about the mode of inheritance are correct:*
   (a) An X-linked inheritance is ruled out if affected fathers have affected sons.

(b) In recessive inheritance, where both parents are known to be carriers, there is a 25% chance that each child will be affected.

(c) In autosomal dominant inheritance, each child of an affected parent has a 50% chance to develop the condition.

(d) A similar prevalence of a particular disorder in both siblings and offspring of an index case strongly supports a probability of an autosomal dominant inheritance.

(e) In polygenic inheritance, environmental factors have no role to play.

5. *The psychometric assessment of personality can be made by using the following tests:*
   (a) The Present State Examination (PSE).
   (b) The Montgomery Asberg Rating Scale.
   (c) The Thematic Apperception Test (TAT).
   (d) The Sentence Completion Test (SCT).
   (e) The Repertory Grid Test.

6. *Imprinting:*
   (a) Is a form of social attachment seen in various species.
   (b) Is known to occur in primates.
   (c) Occurs during the first few months of life.
   (d) Anticipatory anxiety is a common feature.
   (e) It may be related to unacceptable sexual impulses.

7. *The Yerkes-Dodson Curve:*
   (a) Demonstrates the relation between the level of arousal and efficiency of performance.
   (b) Leads to a U-shaped curve.
   (c) Is modified by high levels of anxiety.
   (d) Is primarily concerned with drive and performance.
   (e) Is unaffected by alterations in the level of consciousness.

8. *Primary demyelination occurs in the following neurological disorders:*
   (a) Huntington's chorea.
   (b) Parkinson's disease.
   (c) Wernicke-Korsakoff's syndrome.
   (d) Krabbe's disease.
   (e) Marchiafava-Bignami disease.

9. *The following are important in assessing the effectiveness of a new drug treatment:*
   (a) Placebo wash-out period.
   (b) Constrained randomization.
   (c) Subjective rating scales.
   (d) Placebo control group.
   (e) Cross-over design.

10. *The following disorders occur only in females:*
    (a) Coffin-Lowry syndrome.
    (b) Glucose-6-phosphate dehydrogenase deficiency.
    (c) Aicardi syndrome.
    (d) Niemann-Pick disease.
    (e) Rett syndrome.

11. *An abnormal brain respiratory rate is found in the following conditions:*
    (a) Alzheimer's disease.
    (b) Catatonic stupor.
    (c) Depressive stupor.
    (d) Huntington's chorea.
    (e) Generalized anxiety disorder.

12. *The essential elements of prospective epidemiological studies include:*
    (a) Interviewing the patients' relatives.
    (b) A longitudinal follow-up.
    (c) Random allocation of patients to treatment groups.
    (d) Use of existing case records.
    (e) Psychiatric case registers.

13. *The following disorders are transmitted by a single dominant gene:*
    (a) Cri-du-chat syndrome.
    (b) Acute intermittent porphyria.
    (c) Rett syndrome.
    (d) Acrocallosal syndrome.
    (e) Acrodysostosis.

14. *An abstinence syndrome is known to be caused by the following drugs:*
    (a) Zopiclone.
    (b) Buspirone.
    (c) Caffeine.
    (d) Methaqualone.
    (e) Paroxetine.

15. *Narcissistic defence mechanisms of ego include:*
    (a) Denial.
    (b) Primitive idealization.
    (c) Projective identification.
    (d) Rationalization.
    (e) Reaction formation.

16. *Eye-to-eye contact:*
    (a) Is usually determined by the cultural factors.
    (b) Is one of the essential ingredients of psychotherapy.
    (c) Is influenced by hormonal changes.
    (d) Is reduced in Alzheimer's disease.
    (e) Remains unaffected in depression.

17. *According to the psychoanalytic theory of development of personality, the following statements are correct:*
    (a) There is a minimal importance of genetic factors.
    (b) The development of personality is complete within the first 7 years of life.
    (c) The Oedipus complex occurs in the phallic phase of development.
    (d) Parental guidance is usually considered important in the development of the child.
    (e) Mentally subnormal people have delayed development of their personality.

18. *The following language developmental milestones are correct:*
    (a) Counting up to 10 by 3 years of age.
    (b) Uttering 3 or more words by 18 months of age.
    (c) Giving his or her name by 30 months of age.
    (d) Use of 'mama' and 'dada' by 1 year of age.
    (e) Use of sentences of 4 words by 2½ years of age.

19. *Biofeedback:*
    (a) Is a system which involves an administration of reward and punishment to neurotic patients.
    (b) Is an effective method of modifying cardiovascular functions.
    (c) Involves the provision of information to the patients.
    (d) Is a useful method of conditioning the involuntary autonomic nervous system.
    (e) Teaches the patient to regulate some of the physiological functions.

20. *According to psychoanalytic theory, the mental mechanisms involved in dreams include:*
    (a) Condensation.
    (b) Symbolism.
    (c) Sublimation.
    (d) Rationalization.
    (e) Displacement.

21. *The following disorders are transmitted by a single dominant gene:*
    (a) Huntington's chorea.
    (b) Schizophrenia.
    (c) Alpert syndrome.
    (d) Phenylketonuria.
    (e) Creutzfeldt-Jacob disease.

22. *The rhinencephalon consists of:*
    (a) Fornix.
    (b) Amygdala.
    (c) Olfactory bulbs.
    (d) A strip of paleocortex.
    (e) Olive.

23. *The features of Piaget's preoperational stage include:*
    (a) Circular reaction.
    (b) Law of conservation.
    (c) Precausal reasoning.
    (d) Phenomenalistic causality.
    (e) Animistic thinking.

24. *The standard deviation is a statistical measure of:*
    (a) Statistical significance.
    (b) Frequency.
    (c) Dispersion.
    (d) Variance.
    (e) Departure from the arithmetic mean.

25. *The following statements about standard intelligence tests are correct:*
    (a) They are of little value in people over the age of 65 years.
    (b) They can be modified to meet the special needs of a patient.
    (c) They usually yield normally distributed scores in the general population.
    (d) They can be used universally without any difficulties.
    (e) They are most useful tools in differentiating multi-infarct dementia from other types of dementias.

26. *The following statements about the selective serotonin re-uptake inhibitors are correct:*
    (a) They are extensively eliminated by hepatic metabolism in the form of mostly inactive metabolites.
    (b) Norfluoxetine is an active metabolite of fluoxetine.
    (c) Fluoxetine has a shorter half-life than other compounds which are currently available.
    (d) Wash-out of fluoxetine may take several weeks.
    (e) They have a very small cardiotoxic effect in overdosage.

27. *The characteristic features of parietal lobe lesions include:*
    (a) Visuospatial difficulties.
    (b) Topographic disorientation.
    (c) Anosognosia.

(d) Gerstmann's syndrome.
(e) Agraphaesthesia.

28. *The following statements about carbamazepine are correct:*
(a) It has a three-ringed structure similar to the tricyclic antidepressant drugs.
(b) The commonest side-effects are due to raised plasma concentration.
(c) Allergic rash is a rare side-effect.
(d) Hepatotoxicity is a common side-effect.
(e) Overdosage is frequently fatal.

29. *The characteristic features of attachment behaviour include:*
(a) Crawling or toddling after the mother.
(b) Using mother as a secure base from which to explore the surroundings.
(c) Clinging hard when anxious.
(d) Crying frequently in mother's presence.
(e) Climbing onto mother's lap.

30. *The recognized features of fragile X syndrome include:*
(a) Attention-deficits hyperactivity disorder.
(b) Female carriers are less impaired than males with fragile X.
(c) Small head and ears.
(d) A tall stature.
(e) Post pubertal macro-orchidism.

31. *The neuroglia:*
(a) Are interstitial cells that completely fill the gaps between the nerves.
(b) Are twice the number of neurones.
(c) Are mesodermal in origin.
(d) Form a part of the blood–brain barrier.
(e) Are usually involved in synthesis of neurotransmitters.

32. *The following statements concerning styles of leadership are correct:*
(a) Members of a group with an autocratic leader are aggressive to one another.

(b) Democratic leaders yield greater productivity.
(c) *Laissez-faire* leadership style is good for urgent problems.
(d) Members of a group with a democratic leader abandon the task in the leader's absence.
(e) *Laissez-faire* style is good for creative and original results.

33. *The recognized types of consent include:*
    (a) Express.
    (b) Explicit.
    (c) Implied.
    (d) Oral.
    (e) Valid.

34. *According to the New York longitudinal study, the dimensions of behaviour of young children include:*
    (a) Persistence.
    (b) Aggression.
    (c) Quality of mood.
    (d) Distractability.
    (e) Obstinacy.

35. *The Prion dementias characteristically show:*
    (a) Spongy degeneration of the cerebral grey matter.
    (b) Neuronal proliferation.
    (c) Amyloid protein identical to that seen in Alzheimer's dementia.
    (d) Astrocytic proliferation.
    (e) Lewy bodies in the brain stem.

36. *In comparing Computerized Tomography (CT), Scan with Magnetic Resonance Imaging (MRI):*
    (a) The imaging plane is transverse for CT Scan and vertical for MRI.
    (b) The time taken for both procedures is equal.
    (c) Ionizing radiation is used in the MRI Scan.
    (d) CT Scan is superior in diagnosing demyelinating diseases.
    (e) The basis of tissue contrast in CT Scan is radio density.

37. *The epidemiological studies include:*
    (a) Population survey.
    (b) Double-blind trial.
    (c) Cohort studies.
    (d) Use of case registers.
    (e) Use of hospital morbidity rates.

38. *Conditioned avoidance drive is a manifestation of the neurotic anxiety, which can lead to:*
    (a) Reinforcement of conditioned emotional response.
    (b) Discrimination of conditioned stimuli.
    (c) Elimination of operant behaviour.
    (d) Superstitious behaviour.
    (e) Diminution of the strength of conditioned response.

39. *The following statements about neurotransmitters are correct:*
    (a) The precursor of dopamine is an amino acid with an aromatic side chain.
    (b) The precursor of noradrenaline is an amino acid with a basic side chain.
    (c) The precursor of serotonin is tryptophan.
    (d) Glycine has an aliphatic side chain.
    (e) Glutamate is an amino acid with a basic side chain.

40. *The following statements concerning social class are correct:*
    (a) Social class III has the highest mortality rate for men aged 15 to 64 years.
    (b) Social class I has the lowest mortality rate due to tuberculosis.
    (c) Social class IV has the highest mortality rate due to bronchitis.
    (d) Social class V has the highest rate of chronic illness for men and women.
    (e) Social class II has the fewest number of visits to general practitioners.

41. *The following statements about semantic differentials are correct:*
    (a) They are essentially described as 'forced choice' techniques.

   (b) They are commonly used to measure qualitative aspects of attitudes.

   (c) They are most useful in differentiating schizophrenic thought disorder from non-schizophrenic thought processes.

   (d) Their use involves the use of unipolar adjectival pairs.

   (e) They are not contaminated with the tendency to evoke social desirability in the respondents.

42. *The characteristic features of dominant temporal lobe lesions include:*
   (a) Motor aphasia.
   (b) Severe amnesic syndrome.
   (c) Alexia.
   (d) Agraphia.
   (e) Constructional apraxia.

43. *Down's syndrome:*
   (a) Is the most commonly studied cause of mental retardation.
   (b) Is associated with increased risk of bipolar affective disorder.
   (c) Is associated with an increased risk of further affected children in young mothers with translocation chromosome.
   (d) May be due to increased age of the father.
   (e) Is associated with symptomatic carriers who have only 45 chromosomes.

44. *From the viewpoint of psychoanalysis, the following statements are correct:*
   (a) If children are given adequate sex education, most of the neurotic disorders can be prevented.
   (b) The roots of most adult neurotic problems can be traced to sexual seduction in childhood.
   (c) Negativism is an early-warning feature of adolescent crisis.
   (d) The mother–child relationship during the first year of life is an important factor in determining the child's healthy psychological development.

(e) Countertransference is essential for successful outcome of the therapy.

45. *The ascending white column tracts of the spinal cord include:*
    (a) Posterior spinocerebellar tract.
    (b) Fasciculus cuneatus.
    (c) Tectospinal tract.
    (d) Lateral corticospinal tract.
    (e) Lateral spinothalamic tract.

46. *Drug interactions with carbamazepine include:*
    (a) Increased concentration by cimetidine.
    (b) Decreased concentration by other anticonvulsants.
    (c) Increased concentration by verapamil.
    (d) Decreased metabolism by tricyclic antidepressant compounds.
    (e) Increased metabolism by neuroleptic agents.

47. *Instrumental responses are strengthened by the process of:* (Operant)
    (a) Generalization of the conditioned stimulus.
    (b) Acquisition of autonomic emotional responses.
    (c) Elimination of negative and conditioned stimuli. variable
    (d) Trial and error.
    (e) Reinforcement of their required voluntary behaviour.

48. *The following statements about the phosphoinositide pathway are correct:*
    (a) It is a second messenger pathway.
    (b) It is triggered by enzymatic cleavage of phosphatidylinositol biphosphate.
    (c) The active second messengers are inositol triphosphate (IP3) and inositol tetraphosphate (IP4).
    (d) The compounds inositol triphosphate (IP3) and inositol tetraphosphate (IP4) stimulate a rise in intracellular sodium.
    (e) It may explain the mechanism of action of lithium carbonate.

49. *The observer rated psychiatric instruments include:*
    (a) General Health Questionnaire.
    (b) Leyton Obsessional Inventory.
    (c) Severity of Alcohol Dependence Questionnaire.
    (d) Present State Examination.
    (e) Beck Depression Inventory.

50. *The following statements about the measurement of risk are correct:*
    (a) A value of 1 for the relative risk implies a casual association.
    (b) The odds ratio is useful in prospective studies.
    (c) The attributable risk is also known as the risk difference.
    (d) A value of zero for the attributable risk implies an association.
    (e) The odds ratio is an approximation of the attributable risk.

BASIC SCIENCES
PAPER 2

1. *Cognitive dissonance:*
   (a) Is a concept from social psychology.
   (b) Is a useful concept for cognitive behaviour therapy.
   (c) Is usually not recognized by the subject.
   (d) May be reduced by adding new cognitions which are consonant with pre-existing ones.
   (e) Has been used to analyse different patterns of smoking.

2. *There are significantly more severely subnormal persons than can be accounted for by a chance expectancy at the left-hand side of the intelligence scale. The reasons for this include:*
   (a) Poor socioeconomic status.
   (b) Marital discord.
   (c) Mutation.
   (d) The fact that subnormal people have larger families.
   (e) Perinatal brain injuries.

3. *Psychometric assessment of personality can be made by using the following tests:*
   (a) The Hostility and Direction of the Hostility Questionnaire (HDHQ).
   (b) The General Health Questionnaire (GHQ).
   (c) The Symptom Sign Inventory (SSI).
   (d) The California Psychological Inventory (CPI).
   (e) The Rorschach Inkblot test.

4. *Primary demyelination occurs in the following neurological disorders:*
   (a) Alzheimer's disease.
   (b) Wilson's disease.

(c) Schilder's disease.
(d) Tay-Sachs' disease.
(e) Multiple sclerosis.

5. *The essential features of Piaget's theory of cognitive development include:*
   (a) Basic trust versus mistrust.
   (b) Concrete operational stage.
   (c) Autonomy versus shame and doubt.
   (d) Formal operational stage.
   (e) Sensorimotor stage.

6. *Sampling procedure designed for standardization of Intelligence Quotient (IQ) test involves the following:*
   (a) Socioeconomic status.
   (b) Educational achievements.
   (c) IQ of the parents.
   (d) Chronological age.
   (e) Occupation.

7. *The following disorders occur only in boys:*
   (a) The fragile X syndrome.
   (b) The Lesch-Nyhan syndrome.
   (c) Hunter-Hurler disease.
   (d) Hyperuricaemia.
   (e) Klinefelter's syndrome.

8. *An abnormal brain respiratory rate is found in the following conditions:*
   (a) Multi-infarct dementia.
   (b) Delirium tremens.
   (c) Wernicke's encephalopathy.
   (d) Social phobia.
   (e) Schizophrenia.

9. *According to the psychoanalytic theory of psychosexual development, the fixation at the anal phase is related in adult life to the following:*
   (a) Parsimony.
   (b) Orderliness.

(c) Obstinacy.
(d) Frugality.
(e) Wilfulness.

10. *According to attachment theory:*
    (a) Babies below the age of 6 months do not manifest attachment behaviours.
    (b) Attachment does not occur with people other than the parents.
    (c) Feeding is the key factor in establishing attachment.
    (d) Attachment is formed equally with mother and father.
    (e) Attachment can occur to inanimate objects.

11. *The following disorders are transmitted by a single recessive gene:*
    (a) Down's syndrome.
    (b) Klinefelter's syndrome.
    (c) Hyperprolinaemia types I and II.
    (d) Gaucher's disease.
    (e) Amarotic idiocy.

12. *The following statements about the structures of the cerebral cortex are correct:*
    (a) The primary motor cortex is in the postcentral gyrus of the parietal lobe.
    (b) The primary sensory cortex is in the precentral gyrus of the frontal lobe.
    (c) The visual cortex is in the calcarine fissure of the occipital lobe.
    (d) The auditory cortex is in the uncus and parahippocampal gyrus of the temporal lobe.
    (e) The olfactory cortex is deep within the sylvian fissure in the temporal lobe.

13. *The following statements regarding conditioning experiments are correct:*
    (a) Operant conditioning may be understood in terms of perceptual expectancies.

(b) Intermittent reinforcement in operant conditioning leads to greater resistance to extinction than continuous reinforcement.
(c) Punishment leads to the diminished probability of the occurrence of a response.
(d) Negative reinforcement is synonymous with punishment.
(e) Extinction is the process of gradual disappearance of a conditioned response on discontinuation of an unconditional stimulus.

14. *In dominant occipital lobe lesions, the following are commonly seen:*
(a) Prosopagnosia.
(b) Metamorphosia.
(c) Complex visual hallucinations.
(d) Visuospatial agnosia.
(e) Finger agnosia.

15. *The superego:*
(a) Represents the conscience.
(b) Usually includes unconscious elements.
(c) May be in conflict with present values.
(d) Is an accurate replica of a parental figure in early childhood.
(e) Sometimes overlaps with the ego.

16. *The normal distribution of a variable is important in estimating the following:*
(a) Standard Error of mean.
(b) Variance.
(c) Percentile indices.
(d) A correlation coefficient.
(e) Confidence intervals.

17. *Maternal deprivation frequently results in:*
(a) Development delay in language.
(b) Short stature.
(c) Infantile autism.

   (d) Social disinhibition.
   (e) Shallow relationships with others.

18. *The mature defence mechanisms of ego include:*
   (a) Anticipation.
   (b) Altruism.
   (c) Displacement.
   (d) Sublimation.
   (e) Suppression.

19. *Factor analysis:*
   (a) Is a statistical technique which enables the reduction of the interrelationship within a large sample to a small number of independent factors.
   (b) Was initially formulated by statisticians.
   (c) Has been used successfully to classify psychiatric disorders.
   (d) Assumes that the relationship between the variables and factors is linear.
   (e) Assumes that the variables are liable to random errors.

20. *The following statements about neuroglia are correct:*
   (a) The astrocytes are multipolar cells with several thick processes.
   (b) The glial processes of astrocytes completely cover the outer surfaces of capillaries.
   (c) The oligodendroglia are smaller spherical cells with only a few processes.
   (d) The astrocytes lie in long parallel rows alongside axons.
   (e) The oligodendroglia form the myelin sheath.

21. *Classical conditioning takes place irrespective of:*
   (a) The time interval between conditioned stimulus and unconditioned stimulus.
   (b) The genetic potential of the organism.
   (c) The organism's voluntary behaviour.
   (d) The schedule of reinforcement.
   (e) The nature of the unconditioned stimulus.

22. *It is possible to make a prenatal diagnosis in the following conditions:*
    (a) Huntington's chorea.
    (b) Phenylketonuria.
    (c) Hartnup disorder.
    (d) Niemann-Pick disease, Group A and Group B.
    (e) Galactosaemia.

23. *The features of action potential of a nerve fibre include:*
    (a) Reversal of voltage across the nerve membrane.
    (b) Inward movement of potassium ions.
    (c) Outward movement of chloride ions.
    (d) Inward movement of sodium ions.
    (e) Outward movement of phosphate ions.

24. *The recognized features of difficult, temperamental children include the following:*
    (a) They are irregular in their biological functions.
    (b) They adapt to changes quickly.
    (c) They have a predominantly negative mood.
    (d) There is a three-fold risk factor for subsequent behaviour disorder.
    (e) They have shallow emotional reactions.

25. *The following statements about effects of lithium carbonate on thyroid functioning are correct:*
    (a) Lithium carbonate leads to clinical goitre in the majority of patients.
    (b) Hyperthyroidism is commonly reported.
    (c) Lithium-induced thyroid dysfunction is irreversible.
    (d) Lithium carbonate has to be discontinued if thyroxine is prescribed.
    (e) If thyroid dysfunction does not occur in the first 6 months, monitoring of thyroid functioning can be discontinued.

26. *The G proteins:*
    (a) Are guanine nucleotide binding proteins.
    (b) Are embedded in the cellular membrane.

   (c) Form an intermediate link between a receptor and effector enzymes.

   (d) Are not involved in the adenylate cyclase pathway.

   (e) Are involved as intermediates in receptor-activated ion channels and other post-receptor pathways.

27. *Research has demonstrated the following gender-related differences:*

   (a) Females have better visuospatial differences.

   (b) Males excel in mathematical skills.

   (c) Females have fewer verbal skills.

   (d) Males have better non-verbal skills.

   (e) Females excel in passive aggression.

28. *Mental mechanisms which play an essential part in the production of hysterical conversion symptoms include:*

   (a) Ambivalence.

   (b) Introjection.

   (c) Reaction formation.

   (d) Displacement.

   (e) Denial.

29. *Neuropathological studies of schizophrenia have shown that:*

   (a) The brains of schizophrenic patients are smaller and lighter.

   (b) The frontal horns of their lateral ventricles are larger.

   (c) Most abnormalities are often present in the basal ganglia, hippocampus and parahippocampal gyrus.

   (d) Abnormalities are often prominent on the right side of the brain.

   (e) Changes seen are accompanied by gliosis.

30. *Classical conditioning occurs most efficiently when:*

   (a) The time intervals between conditioned stimulus and unconditioned stimulus are varied.

   (b) Unconditioned stimulus precedes the conditioned stimulus.

   (c) Alternative responses are available for the organism.

(d) Conditioned responses are strengthened by shaping.
(e) The time interval between conditioned stimulus and unconditioned stimulus is fixed at approximately 0.5 seconds.

31. *Lithium-induced neurotoxicity:*
    (a) Is usually irreversible.
    (b) Rarely manifests as pseudotumour cerebri.
    (c) May lead to permanent deficits more often in females than males.
    (d) Is indistinguishable from acute overdose.
    (e) Does not correlate with EEG changes.

32. *Gestalt psychology:*
    (a) States that the properties of some details in a pattern influence how the whole pattern is perceived.
    (b) States that the properties of the whole pattern affect the way the parts are perceived.
    (c) States that the whole is different from the sum of its parts.
    (d) Deals with essential characteristics of actual experience.
    (e) Emphasizes the current experiences of the patient in the here and now.

33. *The components of the basal ganglia include:*
    (a) Insula.
    (b) Globus pallidus.
    (c) Diencephalon.
    (d) Amygdaloid nucleus.
    (e) Claustrum.

34. *In Down's syndrome:*
    (a) There is an extra chromosome 21.
    (b) There is an increased risk of Alzheimer's disease.
    (c) The majority of cases are due to translocation involving chromosome 21.
    (d) The mental retardation is reversible if an early diagnosis is made.
    (e) The life expectancy is comparable to that of the general population.

35. *The characteristic features of GABA receptors include the following:*
   (a) GABA is the main cortical inhibitory neurotransmitter.
   (b) GABA B receptor has a chloride channel that mediates GABAergic transmission.
   (c) Antiepileptic agents act on GABA A receptors.
   (d) GABA receptors are widely distributed with high concentrations in the spinal cord.
   (e) Their functions depend on the presence of GABA transaminase.

36. *The sick role as described by Parsons stipulates that the sick person has:*
   (a) The right to be defined as not responsible for his or her condition.
   (b) The right to take advantage of any secondary gains involved in being sick.
   (c) The right but not the obligation to define the state of being sick as desirable.
   (d) The right to be exempt from normal social activities.
   (e) The option of seeking competent medical help.

37. *To test the hypothesis that two samples are drawn from the same population, an investigator can use the following tests:*
   (a) Factor analysis.
   (b) A chi-square test for independence.
   (c) Principal component analysis.
   (d) Analysis of variance.
   (e) Mann-Whitney U test.

38. *The following statements about the term 'ethology' are correct:*
   (a) It is the study of living organisms in their natural environment.
   (b) It is useful in understanding human non-verbal behaviour.
   (c) It can help in understanding the extrapyramidal speech disorders in human beings.
   (d) It requires a control group for assessment of its effects.
   (e) It is useful in understanding the process of attachment and separation anxiety.

39. *In epidemiological research, the following instruments may be utilized in determining the case level of phenomenology:*
    (a) Feighner criteria.
    (b) General Health Questionnaire.
    (c) Present State Examination.
    (d) Schedule for affective disorders.
    (e) Research diagnostic criteria.

40. *The following phenomena are predictive of an antidepressant effect of a drug:*
    (a) Rapid Eye Movement (REM) sleep latency increase.
    (b) Reserpine antagonism.
    (c) Noradrenaline antagonism.
    (d) Enhancement of chloride channel transmission.
    (e) Selective serotonin re-uptake inhibition.

41. *The following are important models from which observational learning takes place:*
    (a) High status.
    (b) High social class.
    (c) High social power.
    (d) High competence.
    (e) High integrity.

42. *Defence reaction arousal in laboratory animals may be produced by stimulating the following structures in the brain:*
    (a) Hypothalamus.
    (b) Ventrolateral thalamic nucleus.
    (c) Fornix.
    (d) Hippocampus.
    (e) Globus pallidus.

43. *In clinical research, the samples may be selected by using the following techniques:*
    (a) Stratification.
    (b) Multiphasic.
    (c) Double-blind.
    (d) Multistage.
    (e) Minimization.

44. *The principles of the Gestalt school of perception include:*
    (a) Law of closure.
    (b) Law of continuity.
    (c) Law of infinity.
    (d) Law of proximity.
    (e) Law of similarity.

45. *The characteristic features of calcium channels in the neurones include the following:*
    (a) Neurotransmitter release usually depends on calcium.
    (b) Calcium channels close in response to membrane depolarization.
    (c) There is only one type of calcium channel known to occur in the neurones.
    (d) Some of the side-effects of the neuroleptic drugs are due to calcium channel blockade.
    (e) Channel blockers like nifedipine and verapamil influence neurotransmitter release.

46. *The most effective methods of reducing racial prejudice include:*
    (a) Improving the image of ethnic minorities in the media.
    (b) Psychotherapy for black–white confrontations.
    (c) Interracial contact.
    (d) Introducing the studies of ethnic groups into the school curriculum.
    (e) Legislating against discriminative behaviour.

47. *The characteristic features of Down's syndrome include:*
    (a) Congenital cardiac disease.
    (b) Brushfield spots.
    (c) A single transverse palmar crease.
    (d) Bradycephaly.
    (e) Umbilical hernias.

48. *The placebo reaction in clinical drug trials:*
    (a) Refers to the patient's tendency to react to the colour, shape and size of the drug preparation.

   (b) Refers to the patient's tendency to describe side-effects on the basis of expectancy and mental attitudes even to dummy preparations.

   (c) Can be influenced by a side-effects questionnaire.

   (d) Refers to the tendency to improve within the first 2 weeks of treatment.

   (e) Depends on the seniority of the prescriber.

49. *The following statements about benzodiazepine dependence are correct:*

   (a) There is a considerable evidence for genetic predisposition in some patients.

   (b) The clinical picture is characteristically different from heroin addiction.

   (c) The mechanism for persistent withdrawal symptoms is well understood.

   (d) Ventricular enlargement on CT Scan has been consistent in long-term benzodiazepine users.

   (e) It is associated with a specific personality structure.

50. *The following statements concerning reinforcement in operant conditioning are correct:*

   (a) Variable ratio reinforcement is the easiest to extinguish.

   (b) Intermittent reinforcement takes the longest to establish.

   (c) Fixed ratio reinforcement involves reinforcing after a fixed interval of time of continuous response.

   (d) Secondary reinforcement involves natural reinforcement through decrease of basic drive.

   (e) Negative reinforcement can mean reinforcement through withdrawal of unpleasant conditions.

BASIC SCIENCES
PAPER 3

1. *The functions of neuroglia include the following:*
   - (a) Astrocytes help to form the blood–brain barrier.
   - (b) Microglia are phagocytic.
   - (c) Astrocytes are involved in phagocytosis.
   - (d) Schwann cells form the myelin sheath of central neurones.
   - (e) Ependyma cells line the central canal of the spinal cord.

2. *The statistical significant association at P = 0.05 between two variables implies:*
   - (a) That a cause-and-effect relationship is established.
   - (b) That approximately 95% of the variance has been accounted for in this particular experiment.
   - (c) An association likely to occur by chance only in 5 out of 100 cases.
   - (d) Measurements of proven validity and reliability.
   - (e) That data are trustworthy and useful.

3. *The following disorders occur only in males:*
   - (a) Cerebellar ataxia.
   - (b) Phenylketonuria.
   - (c) Gaucher's disease.
   - (d) X-linked hydrocephalus.
   - (e) The W-syndrome.

4. *According to Freud's theory of psychosexual development, the fixation at the oral stage is related in adult life to the following:*
   - (a) Narcissism.
   - (b) Stubbornness.
   - (c) Excessive optimism.
   - (d) Pessimism.
   - (e) 'Identity diffusion'.

5. *Cognitive dissonance:*
   (a) Arises when there is palpable disparity between 2 behavioural elements.
   (b) When resolved, leads to decreased internal discomfort.
   (c) Results in self-deception.
   (d) Is usually found in schizophrenia.
   (e) Leads to attitude change.

6. *The essential features of Erik Erikson's theory of psychosocial development include:*
   (a) Separation anxiety.
   (b) Initiative versus guilt.
   (c) Industry versus inferiority.
   (d) Preoperational stage.
   (e) Identity versus role confusion.

7. *Defence reaction arousal in laboratory animals may be produced by stimulating the following structures in the brain:*
   (a) Cingulate gynis.
   (b) Stria terminalis.
   (c) Anterior thalamus.
   (d) Dentate gyrus.
   (e) Amygdaloid body.

8. *Examination of the buccal smear for sex chromatin (Barr Bodies) is of diagnostic value in the following disorders:*
   (a) XXY syndrome.
   (b) XYY syndrome.
   (c) Wilson's disease.
   (d) Hartnup disease.
   (e) Edward's syndrome.

9. *The characteristic microscopic findings of Alzheimer's disease include:*
   (a) Plaques which are composed of paired helical filaments.
   (b) Tangles which consist of amyloid precursor protein deposits.
   (c) Hirano bodies which are eosinophilic cigar-shaped bodies.

   (d) Cellular loss in the basal magnocellular nucleus of Meynert.
   (e) Amyloid deposition in the ventricular walls.

10. *The extrinsic motivation theories include the following:*
   (a) Needs activate drives.
   (b) Drive reduction has reinforcing properties for learning a behaviour.
   (c) Needs originate from biological homeostasis.
   (d) Needs arise out of physiological homeostatic imbalance.
   (e) Secondary drives are acquired by learning.

11. *The Standard Error is a measure of:*
   (a) Central tendency.
   (b) The most frequent observation.
   (c) Range of observations.
   (d) The mean of the population.
   (e) Robustness of the experiment.

12. *The recognized causes of subcortical dementia include:*
   (a) Wilson's disease.
   (b) Huntington's disease.
   (c) AIDS dementia complex.
   (d) Normal pressure hydrocephalus.
   (e) Parkinson's disease.

13. *Piaget's preoperational stage includes the following:*
   (a) Characteristic egocentrism.
   (b) Mastery of conservation.
   (c) Rules are inviolate.
   (d) Ability to detach logic from immediate experience.
   (e) Animism.

14. *The following disorders are transmitted by a single recessive gene:*
   (a) Fragile X syndrome.
   (b) Lesch-Nyhan syndrome.
   (c) Coffin-Lowry syndrome.
   (d) Bipolar affective disorder.
   (e) Patau's syndrome.

15. *The branches of the Circle of Willis include:*
    (a) Middle cerebral artery.
    (b) Anterior choroidal artery.
    (c) Ophthalmic artery.
    (d) Anterior inferior cerebellar artery.
    (e) Posterior communicating artery.

16. *The following statements about drug activity and neuroreceptors are correct:*
    (a) The drugs that bind to receptors and initiate a response are agonists.
    (b) The drugs that produce a response opposite to the normal response after binding to receptors are antagonists.
    (c) Some drugs are known to have both agonist and antagonist activity.
    (d) Reverse agonists are drugs that produce effects by preventing an agonist from initiating a response.
    (e) Affinity refers to the ease with which a drug attaches to a receptor.

17. *The unified theory of Maslow involves:*
    (a) Love and belonging.
    (b) Competence.
    (c) Autonomy.
    (d) Curiosity.
    (e) Self-esteem.

18. *The following are recognized features of adolescence:*
    (a) Puberty occurs earlier in boys.
    (b) Adolescent turmoil is considered to be essential to healthy adolescent development.
    (c) Adolescents rarely identify with their parents' values.
    (d) Acquisition of formal operational thought occurs in adolescence.
    (e) School-aged adolescents tend to be mainly groups of the same sex.

19. *It is possible to make a prenatal diagnosis in the following conditions:*
    (a) Hunter's syndrome.
    (b) Wilson's hepatolenticular degeneration.
    (c) Tay-Sachs' disease.
    (d) Krabbe's disease.
    (e) Niemann-Pick disease.

20. *The neuropathology of multiple sclerosis shows:*
    (a) That plaques develop along the course of small veins.
    (b) That disruption of the blood–brain barrier occurs.
    (c) White matter changes as seen on Magnetic Resonance Imaging (MRI) occur only in periventricular areas.
    (d) Astrocytic gliosis.
    (e) Predominant lesions in the white matter of the brain.

21. *The measures of central tendency of distribution include:*
    (a) Median.
    (b) Mode.
    (c) Average.
    (d) Quartiles.
    (e) Range.

22. *Ethnic differences in response to pain are attributable mainly to:*
    (a) Experimental bias.
    (b) Intellectual ability to understand the significance of disease.
    (c) Differences in subjective experience of pain.
    (d) Cultural stoicism or emotionalism.
    (e) Differences in tolerance threshold.

23. *The following statements about diagnostic interviews are correct:*
    (a) The Present State Examination (PSE) provides operational definition of each symptom to be rated.
    (b) The Present State Examination (PSE) provides no criteria for severity.
    (c) The Present State Examination (PES) can be used to characterize illnesses.

(d) The American version of PSE is called the SADS (Schedule for Affective Disorders and Schizophrenia).
(e) The SADS is identical to the PSE in the scope of application.

24. *Statistically significant association between two variables implies that:*
    (a) A cause-and-effect relationship has certainly been established.
    (b) The measurements are of proven reliability and validity.
    (c) 95% of the variance has been accounted for.
    (d) The association is likely to occur by chance only at a stated low level of probability.
    (e) The p value is >0.001.

25. *The stimulation of dopamine receptors characteristically causes:*
    (a) Tardive dyskinesia.
    (b) Acute dystonic reactions.
    (c) Sedation.
    (d) Nausea and vomiting.
    (e) Excitement.

26. *The immature defence mechanisms of ego include:*
    (a) Identification.
    (b) Inhibition.
    (c) Intellectualization.
    (d) Introjection.
    (e) Isolation.

27. *The following statements about matching in epidemiological studies are correct:*
    (a) Most commonly the comparison group does not differ from the study group with regard to the diagnosis.
    (b) The comparison group is matched according to the main features of the study group.
    (c) The matched group eliminates unwanted variables.
    (d) Matching can eliminate more variables than the investigator intends.

(e) The matched group is normally a random sample from the population from which it is drawn.

28. *The following antipsychotic drugs are correctly paired with their drug class:*
    (a) Droperidol – thioxanthene.
    (b) Pimozide – diphenylbutylpiperidine.
    (c) Clozapine – dibenzoxazepine.
    (d) Prochlorperazine – phenothiazine.
    (e) Risperidone – butyrophenone.

29. *The features of the measurement instruments of attitude include the following:*
    (a) The Thurstone Scale is a 5-point scale where the subject is presented with a number of statements.
    (b) In the Likert Scale the subject is presented with a range of statements on which he or she ticks those agreed with.
    (c) The Likert Scale is more sensitive than the Thurstone scale.
    (d) Semantic differential is where a series of two evaluative adjectives or verbs, each at either end of a line, act as a visual analogue scale.
    (e) Lie scales are used to counter the problem of social desirability set answers.

30. *Psychotropic drugs produce the following EEG changes:*
    (a) Benzodiazepine drugs show an increase in fast beta activity.
    (b) Lithium carbonate is associated with diffuse slowing.
    (c) Monoamine oxidase inhibitors have a slight effect on the electroencephalogram.
    (d) Tricyclic antidepressant agents show an increase in delta and theta activity.
    (e) Lithium carbonate shows disorganization of background rhythm.

31. *The requirements of psychosurgery in the United Kingdom include:*
    (a) Informed consent from the patient's next of kin.

(b) Independent assessment by an approved doctor and two lay persons that the patient is capable of giving consent.
(c) Compulsory detention under the Mental Health Act.
(d) A diagnosis of intractable generalized anxiety disorder.
(e) Absence of psychopathy.

32. *Optic chiasma:*
    (a) Is situated anterior to the pituitary stalk.
    (b) Is situated lateral to the internal carotid artery.
    (c) Is a cross-junction of both sensory and motor nerve fibres.
    (d) Receives axons from the bipolar cells of the retina.
    (e) Is responsible for the bilateral vision in both eyes.

33. *The excitatory amino acid neurotransmitters:*
    (a) Include glutamate and aspartate.
    (b) Act on the NMDA receptors.
    (c) Act on the kainite and guisqualate receptors.
    (d) Play an important role in learning and memory.
    (e) Are found to lead to hyperpolarization in neurones.

34. *The characteristic features of Poisson distribution include the following:*
    (a) It is a unimodal type of distribution.
    (b) It requires the events to occur randomly in space or time.
    (c) The mean number of events per given unit of time or space is constant.
    (d) It requires the events to occur simultaneously.
    (e) The sum of corresponding probabilities is one.

35. *The following names are linked with idiographic theories of personality:*
    (a) Eysenck.
    (b) Kelly.
    (c) Cattell.
    (d) Rogers.
    (e) Reich.

36. *The following statements about the energy metabolism of the brain include the following:*
    (a) The brain can utilize lipids and protein for energy.
    (b) The brain has large stores of glycogen.
    (c) Under special circumstances the brain can utilize ketone bodies for energy.
    (d) The brain differs from other tissues because of increased activity of the 'GABA Shunt' pathway.
    (e) The cerebral metabolic rate declines in Alzheimer's disease.

37. *The essential features of benzodiazepine withdrawal syndrome include:*
    (a) Increased sensory perception.
    (b) Anxiety.
    (c) Headache.
    (d) Depersonalization.
    (e) Anorexia.

38. *The Cohort Studies:*
    (a) Include defined groups of individuals studied over a period of time.
    (b) Can only be prospective.
    (c) Include changes in the population due to age, which must be distinguished from the disease process.
    (d) Are affected by period effects.
    (e) Provide valuable information on the nature of a relationship between groups.

39. *The following concepts in ethology have made significant contributions to the understanding of human behaviour:*
    (a) Imprinting.
    (b) Critical period.
    (c) Fixed action pattern.
    (d) Ethnic bonds.
    (e) 'Sign stimulus'.

40. *Lithium-induced neurotoxicity:*
    (a) Can occur during maintenance therapy.

(b) Can occur with serum lithium level within therapeutic range.
(c) Is usually precipitated by restricted fluid intake.
(d) Results in persisting neurological sequelae in some cases.
(e) Leads to unique EEG changes.

41. *The following statements about sleep are correct:*
    (a) In neonates, REM sleep represents more than 50% of total sleep time.
    (b) Most of the human growth hormone is secreted during REM sleep.
    (c) Slow-wave sleep shows decreased metabolic rate.
    (d) Benzodiazepine drugs suppress slow-wave sleep.
    (e) Tricyclic antidepressant drugs suppress REM sleep.

42. *The geometric mean:*
    (a) Is the reciprocal of the harmonic mean.
    (b) Is the square root of the products of more than 2 observations.
    (c) Should be used in preference to the arithmetic mean in dealing with sensitive data.
    (d) Is computed by dividing the coefficient of variation by the standard deviation.
    (e) Is more representative than the arithmetic mean in very skewed observations.

43. *According to the recent knowledge about dopamine receptors:*
    (a) D2 receptors are coupled to adenylate cyclase.
    (b) Two forms of D2 receptors have been identified.
    (c) D3 and D4 receptors have also been described.
    (d) D2 receptor is coupled to G proteins.
    (e) D1 receptors are found in abundance in the pituitary gland.

44. *Research on medical students' psychiatric interview techniques reveal that:*
    (a) They enthusiastically elicit the sexual history.
    (b) They frequently interrupt patients.

(c) They are often afraid to look at a watch or clock in case this upsets patients.

(d) Jargon is usually accepted from patients.

(e) Non-verbal cues are usually picked up.

45. *The characteristic features of new-born infants suffering from Down's syndrome include:*
   (a) Generalized hypertonia.
   (b) A small tongue.
   (c) Oblique palpebral fissures.
   (d) A small, flattened skull.
   (e) High cheek bones.

46. *The following statements about the blood–brain barrier are correct:*
   (a) Proteins readily enter the brain through the blood–brain barrier.
   (b) Lipid-soluble substances pass slowly into the brain.
   (c) It regulates the movement of substances into and out of the brain.
   (d) It is facilitated by gaps between the cells of capillary endothelium.
   (e) It is only a functional rather than an actual barrier.

47. *The following statements about cognitive dissonance are correct:*
   (a) It deals with people striving for consistency between cognitions thought by them to be related.
   (b) Dissonance can arise out of conflicting expectations.
   (c) Dissonance is experienced as uncomfortable and leads to attempts to reduce it.
   (d) The less important the cognitions, the more powerful the dissonance.
   (e) Dissonance may be reduced by dismissing information creating dissonance.

48. *The characteristic features of Type A personality include:*
   (a) Extreme competitiveness.
   (b) Need for peer approval.
   (c) Explosiveness of speech.

    (d)   Reduced rate of myocardial infarction.
    (e)   Striving for achievement.

49.   *Benzodiazepines may cause the following side-effects in therapeutic dosages:*
    (a)   Anterograde amnesia.
    (b)   Ataxia.
    (c)   Blurred vision.
    (d)   Maculopapular rashes.
    (e)   Nausea.

50.   *Complete or partial occlusion of the following arteries are paired correctly with their deficits:*
    (a)   Posterior cerebral artery – alexia without agraphia.
    (b)   Anterior cerebral artery – contralateral paresis of upper limb only.
    (c)   Middle cerebral artery – contralateral hemianopsia.
    (d)   Basilar artery – locked-in syndrome.
    (e)   Posterior inferior cerebellar artery – Horner's syndrome.

BASIC SCIENCES
ANSWERS TO
PAPER 1

1. (a) T.
   (b) F.
   (c) F.
   (d) T.
   (e) T.
   It occurs when there is a palpable discrepancy between 2 experimental or behavioural elements. It is not confined to any specific diagnostic categories.

2. (a) F. Projective identification allows one to distance and make oneself understood by exerting pressure on another person to experience feelings similar to one's own.
   (b) T.
   (c) T.
   (d) T.
   (e) T.

3. (a) F. Sodomy is sexual intercourse with a dead body.
   (b) F. Freud viewed homosexuality as an arrest in psychosexual development. He believed that female homosexuality was due to a lack of resolution of penis envy in association with unresolved Oedipal conflicts.
   (c) T.
   (d) F. Bestiality is the use of an animal as a repeated and preferred or exclusive method of achieving sexual excitement.
   (e) T.

4. (a) T. In X-linked inheritance, male-to-male transmission does not occur.
   (b) T. One in 4 children are affected.
   (c) T.
   (d) T.
   (e) F. Environmental factors have an important role to play in various types of inheritance, including polygenic inheritance.

5. (a) F. It is useful in assessing symptoms of psychotic patients.
   (b) F. It is useful in rating the severity of depression.
   (c) T. A projective test.
   (d) T. A projective test.
   (e) T. It is useful in revealing characteristics of neurotic patients.

6. (a) T.
   (b) F. There is no evidence that it occurs in primates.
   (c) T. It is a special form of learning quite different from ordinary conditioning. It is limited to a very brief period, fixed soon after birth, and it is irreversible.
   (d) T.
   (e) F.

7. (a) T.
   (b) F. An inverted, U-shaped curve.
   (c) T.
   (d) T.
   (e) F.

8. (a) F. Neuronal loss in cerebral cortex, particularly affecting the frontal lobes, and in the corpus striatum of basal ganglia.
   (b) F. There is depigmentation and neuronal loss of substantia nigra, particularly of the zona compacta.
   (c) F. Secondary demyelination due to severe deficiency of thiamin (vitamin B1).
   (d) F. Due to deficiency of enzyme galacto-cerebroside B galactosidase, which leads to secondary demyelination.

(e) F. Caused by chronic alcoholism. There is a
widespread demyelination in the brain.

9. (a) T. It is necessary to identify placebo responders and
also patients whose illness remits spontaneously.
(b) T. It ensures that a certain number of patients have
been entered in similar proportions in each
treatment group.
(c) T.
(d) T. It is one of the most important requirements,
during initial assessment of a new drug.
(e) F. It is not helpful in clinical trials of a new drug but in
assessing treatment differences within the same
subjects.

10. (a) F.
(b) F.
(c) F.
(d) F.
(e) F.
When an affected male mates with an unaffected female, all
the daughters and none of the sons will be affected. When
an affected heterozygous female mates with an unaffected
male, on average half of sons and daughters will be affected.

11. (a) T.
(b) F.
(c) F.
(d) T.
(e) F.

12. (a) F. Useful in retrospective study.
(b) T.
(c) F.
(d) F. An element of retrospective study.
(e) T.

13. (a) F. It is caused by a partial deletion of the short arm of
chromosome 5.
(b) T. It is also known as porphobilinogen deaminase
deficiency, or the Swedish type of porphyria.

   (c) T. Mutation on X-chromosome presenting with characteristic deterioration of hand skills and stereotyped hand movements.

   (d) T. It is characterized by absence of corpus callosum, macrocephaly and severe mental retardation.

   (e) T. It is characterized by alopecia, psychomotor epilepsy, pyorrhoea and mental subnormality.

14. (a) F.
   (b) F.
   (c) T.
   (d) T.
   (e) F.
There are anecdotal reports of withdrawal symptoms after short administration of zopidone and buspirone. However, there is a strong suspicion that an abstinence syndrome may occur following a prolonged administration.

15. (a) T.
   (b) T.
   (c) T.
   (d) F. It is a neurotic defence mechanism.
   (e) F. It is a neurotic defence mechanism.

16. (a) T.
   (b) T.
   (c) F.
   (d) T.
   (e) F. Downcast eyes with vertical furrows on the brow with a slight raising of the medial aspect of each eyebrow.

17. (a) F.
   (b) F.
   (c) T.
   (d) F.
   (e) F.
According to psychoanalytic theory, our personalities are basically determined by inborn drives and environmental influences in the first 5 years of life.

Sigmund Freud believed that the personality is composed of 3 major systems that interact to govern human behaviour: the id, the ego and the superego.

18. (a) F.
    (b) T.
    (c) T.
    (d) T.
    (e) F.
The child can count up to 10 by age 4 and use the sentences of 4 words by age 3.

19. (a) F.
    (b) T.
    (c) T.
    (d) T.
    (e) T.
Biofeedback is the application of operant conditioning in which human subjects are given feedback on their autonomic nervous system functioning or motor function and are taught to exert some control over it.

20. (a) T.
    (b) T.
    (c) F.
    (d) F.
    (e) T.
It is gratification of a socially unacceptable impulse by changing into a socially valued one. Sublimation of aggressive impulses takes place through pleasurable games and sports. Rationalization is a justification of attitudes, belief or behaviour that may otherwise be unacceptable by an incorrect application of justifying reasons.

21. (a) T.
    (b) F.
    (c) T.
    (d) F.
    (e) F.
Huntington's chorea and Alpert's syndrome are autosomal

dominant disorders. Phenylketomuria is an autosomal recessive disorder requiring two abnormal alleles. Schizophrenia and Creutzfeldt-Jacob disease do not seem to follow Mendel's laws of inheritance.

22. (a) F.
    (b) F.
    (c) T.
    (d) T.
    (e) F.
The fornix and the amygdala are part of the limbic system. The olive is a part of the medulla oblongata.

23. (a) F.
    (b) F.
    (c) T.
    (d) T.
    (e) T.
Circular reaction occurs in the sensorimotor stage, while the law of conservation occurs in the concrete operational stage of cognitive development.

24. (a) F.
    (b) F.
    (c) T.
    (d) F.
    (e) T.
Statistical significance is measured by different tests like the t-test. Frequency distribution is a systematic way of arranging data. Variance is a measure arrived at by squaring all the deviations, summing them up and then dividing them by the numbers of measures.

25. (a) F.
    (b) T.
    (c) T.
    (d) F.
    (e) F.
The standard intelligence tests are useful in elderly people. As they are in English, translations into other languages may not be accurate.

26. (a) T.
    (b) T.
    (c) F. After chronic administration, the elimination half-life of fluoxetine is about 8 days, while other compounds have a shorter half-life.
    (d) T. Norfluoxetine, an active metabolite has an elimination half-life of about 20 days; hence a period of several weeks is required before the drug is washed out. Thus a caution is necessary when prescribing drugs that interact with fluoxetine.
    (e) F. The current knowledge suggests that these compounds have clinically and pharmacologically non-significant cardiotoxic effect in therapeutic dosages. However, they do have some cardiovascular effects in an overdosage, which are non-fatal.

27. (a) T.
    (b) T.
    (c) T. Anosognosia refers to lack of awareness of disease.
    (d) T.
    (e) T. Agraphaesthesia refers to inability to name figures written on the hand.

28. (a) T.
    (b) T.
    (c) F. It consists of raised red, patchy skin lesions which occur in 12–15% of psychiatrically ill patients.
    (d) F. It is a rare side-effect.
    (e) F. Fatal overdosage is very rare.

29. (a) T.
    (b) T.
    (c) T.
    (d) F.
    (e) T.

30. (a) T.
    (b) T.
    (c) F. Usually large head and ears and short stature.
    (d) F.
    (e) T.

31. (a) T.
    (b) F.
    (c) F.
    (d) T.
    (e) F.
    The neuroglia are about 5 to 10 times the number of
    neurones and are ectodermal in origin.

32. (a) T.
    (b) T.
    (c) F. An autocratic style of leadership is good for solving
        urgent problems.
    (d) F.
    (e) T.

33. (a) T.
    (b) F.
    (c) T.
    (d) T.
    (e) T.

34. (a) T.
    (b) F.
    (c) T.
    (d) T.
    (e) F.
    A total of nine dimensions of behaviour were identified
    including activity level, rhythmicity of biological functions,
    approach/withdrawal to novelty, adaptability, threshold of
    responsiveness to stimuli, and intensity of reaction.

35. (a) T.
    (b) F.
    (c) F.
    (d) T.
    (e) F.
    The Prion dementias in human beings are represented by
    Creutzfeldt-Jacob's disease, Gerstmann-Straussler
    syndrome and Kuru. As neurones cannot regenerate, there
    can be no neuronal proliferation. Lewy bodies in the brain
    stem are characteristic of Parkinson's disease.

36. (a) F. The imaging plane is tranverse for both procedures.
    (b) F. The MRI takes twice as much time as the CT Scan.
    (c) F. While ionizing radiation is used in the CT Scan, none is used in the MRI.
    (d) F. The MRI is in fact superior to the CT Scan.
    (e) T.

37. (a) T.
    (b) F. It is not an epidemiological study but a method of reducing bias in a research study.
    (c) T.
    (d) T.
    (e) T.

38. (a) T.
    (b) T.
    (c) F.
    (d) T.
    (e) F.

39. (a) T.
    (b) F.
    (c) T.
    (d) T.
    (e) F.

40. (a) F.
    (b) T.
    (c) F.
    (d) T.
    (e) F.
    Social class studies reveal that those in class V have the highest rates of disease and the most visits to general practitioners.

41. (a) T.
    (b) F.
    (c) F.
    (d) F.
    (e) T.

42. (a) F. It is caused by lesions in Broca's area.
    (b) F. It results from bilateral lesions of the medial temporal lobe structures.
    (c) T. Caused by posterior lesions of the temporal lobe.
    (d) T. As above.
    (e) T.

43. (a) T.
    (b) F.
    (c) T.
    (d) T.
    (e) T.
    It is associated with an increased risk of Alzheimer's disease in the relatives of the patient.

44. (a) F.
    (b) F.
    (c) F.
    (d) T.
    (e) F.
    Mild anxiety depression and minor disagreement with authority figures are early signs of adolescent crisis. Countertransference can be an impediment but it can be turned into an advantage.

45. (a) T.
    (b) T.
    (c) F.
    (d) F.
    (e) T.
    Tectospinal and lateral corticospinal tracts are not ascending tracts.

46. (a) T.
    (b) T.
    (c) T.
    (d) F.
    (e) T.

47. (a) F.
    (b) F.
    (c) F.
    (d) T.
    (e) T.

48. (a) T. It is linked to a number of membrane-bound
           receptors through an intermediate G protein.
    (b) T.
    (c) T.
    (d) F. The activation leads to an increase in intracellular
           calcium.
    (e) T.

49. (a) F. Self-rating scales.
    (b) F.
    (c) F.
    (d) T.
    (e) F. Self-rating scales.

50. (a) F. The relative risk of a disease with respect to a given
           risk factor is the ratio of the incidence of the disease
           in people exposed to the incidence of the disease in
           the people not exposed. A value of relative risk
           implies no causation.
    (b) F.
    (c) T. The attributable risk is the incidence of the disease
           in the group exposed to the risk factor minus the
           incidence of the group not exposed. A value of zero
           for attributable risk implies no association.
    (d) F.
    (e) T.

1. (a) T.
   (b) T. Cognitive behaviour therapy aims at a primary change in cognition followed by a secondary change in behaviour.
   (c) T.
   (d) T.
   (e) T.

2. (a) T.
   (b) F.
   (c) F.
   (d) F.
   (e) T.
   Large families have more subnormal children than their fair share, but subnormal people do not necessarily have large families.

3. (a) T. Self-report of medical patients with symptoms of anxiety or depression.
   (b) F. It allows measurement of 18 traits that are part of normal personality, such as achievement, sociability, etc.
   (c) F.
   (d) T.
   (e) T. A projective test which involves a number of inkblots none of which has any definite meaning.

4. (a) F. Global atrophy of the brain mainly due to neuronal loss, shrinkage of dendritic branding and a reactive astrocytosis in the cerebral cortex.

(b) F. The main changes are widespread copper deposition in the central nervous system, particularly marked in the basal ganglia.
(c) T.
(d) F. It is due to deficiency of the enzyme N-acetyl-B-hexosaminidase, which may lead to secondary demyelination.
(e) T.

5. (a) F. It is the first stage of psychosocial development of a child as proposed by Erik Erikson.
   (b) T. It is the stage occurring between the ages of 7 and 12 years.
   (c) F. This is the stage in the psychosocial development of the child occurring between the ages of 1 and 3 years.
   (d) T. This is the last stage, which occurs from the age of 12 years onwards.
   (e) T. This is the first stage of the child's cognitive development.

6. (a) T.
   (b) T.
   (c) F.
   (d) T.
   (e) T.
   The intelligence quotient (IQ) is the ratio of mental age over chronological age multiplied by 100 doing away with the decimal point. IQ is a measure of present functioning ability, not necessarily of future potential.

7. (a) T. Female carriers of fragile X syndrome may manifest the typical physical characteristics; e.g. large head and ears; a long, narrow face; short stature; and post-pubertal macro-orchidism.
   (b) T.
   (c) T.
   (d) T.
   (e) T.

8. (a) T.
   (b) T.
   (c) T.
   (d) F.
   (e) F.

9. (a) T.
   (b) T.
   (c) T.
   (d) T.
   (e) T.

10. (a) T.
    (b) F. The attachment is the baby's special relationship with significant primary care givers. It starts developing during the first months after birth. The infant is capable of multiple attachments.
    (c) F.
    (d) T.
    (e) T.

11. (a) F. It is the commonest autosomal abnormality of trisomy 21 due to non-disjunction and translocation.
    (b) F. It is a sex chromosome abnormality in which phenotypic males possess more than one X-chromosome per somatic cell nucleus.
    (c) T.
    (d) T.
    (e) T.

12. (a) F.
    (b) F.
    (c) T.
    (d) F.
    (e) F.
    Answer (a) is true for answer (b), and vice versa. Answer (d) is true for answer (e), and vice versa.

13. (a) F.
    (b) T.
    (c) T. Punishment is an aversive stimulus which is presented specifically to reduce the probability that response will recur.
    (d) F. Negative reinforcement is an aversive stimulus the removal of which increases the probability of occurrence of operant behaviour.
    (e) T.

14. (a) F. It is an ability to recognize known faces.
    (b) F. It is a distortion of objects.
    (c) F.
    (d) F.
    (e) F. Seen in Gerstmann's syndrome and dominant parietal lobe lesions.

15. (a) F.
    (b) F.
    (c) T.
    (d) F.
    (e) T.
    The superego comes into being with the resolution of the Oedipus complex, which leads to a rapid acceleration of the identification process with the parent of the same sex. The identification is based on the child's struggles to repress the instinctual aims. This effort of renunciation gives the super-ego its prohibiting character.

16. (a) T.
    (b) T.
    (c) T.
    (d) T.
    (e) T.

17. (a) T.
    (b) T.
    (c) F. Children suffering from infantile autism resemble emotionally deprived children, but there are distinguishing features in clinical presentation; e.g.

abnormalities in play, stereotypes, ritualistic
behaviours, insistence on sameness and resistance to
change.
(d) T.
(e) T.

18. (a) T.
    (b) T.
    (c) F. It is a neurotic defence mechanism.
    (d) T.
    (e) T.

19. (a) T.
    (b) F. It was formulated by psychologists.
    (c) T.
    (d) T.
    (e) T.

20. (a) T.
    (b) T.
    (c) T. The oligodendroglia lie in long parallel rows
            alongside axons.
    (d) F.
    (e) T.

21. (a) F. The time relationship between the presentation of
            the conditioned and unconditioned stimuli is
            important, varying for optimal learning from a
            fraction of a second to several seconds. Classical
            conditioning is most often applied to responses
            mediated by the autonomic nervous system. The
            reinforcement schedule is required in operant
            conditioning.
    (b) T.
    (c) T.
    (d) F.
    (e) F.

22. (a) T. It is transmitted as an autosomal dominant gene on the G8 fragment of chromosome 4.
    (b) F. Defect of phenylalanine hydroxylase.
    (c) F. A renal transport disorder.
    (d) T. Defect of sphingomyelinase.
    (e) T. Defect of galactose-1-phosphate uridyltransferase.

23. (a) T.
    (b) F.
    (c) F.
    (d) T.
    (e) F.
    An action potential is a self-propagating transmembrane current that occurs when the intraneuronal electrical potential reaches its threshold. Movement of potassium ions out of the membrane increases. The chloride and phosphate ions are not involved in the action potential. The passage of action potential along a neuronal axon is an all-or-nothing phenomenon.

24. (a) T.
    (b) F.
    (c) T.
    (d) T.
    (e) F.
    10% of the children in the New York longitudinal study were categorized as having a difficult temperament. They are negative, slow to adapt to changes, show withdrawal reactions to novelty and have intense emotional reactions.

25. (a) F. Thyroid goitre occurs in a small percentage of patients.
    (b) F. It is very rare, suggesting a possibility that cases may be coincidental.
    (c) F.
    (d) F. Thyroxine can be prescribed, together with lithium carbonate.
    (e) F. All patients on lithium require monitoring of thyroid functions at least annually.

26. (a) T.
    (b) T.
    (c) T.
    (d) F.
    (e) T.
    The G proteins are so named because they require
    guanosine triphosphate (GTP) for their action. They are
    sometimes referred to as the N proteins for nucleotide-
    binding regulatory protein. They affect the activity of
    adenylate cyclase, which, when active, converts adenosine
    triphosphate (ATP) into cyclic-AMP.

27. (a) F.
    (b) T.
    (c) F.
    (d) F.
    (e) T.

28. (a) F.
    (b) F.
    (c) F.
    (d) F.
    (e) F.
    According to psychoanalytic theory, conversion is caused
    by repression of unconscious intra-psychic conflict and the
    conversion of the anxiety into a physical symptom.

29. (a) T.
    (b) F.
    (c) T.
    (d) F.
    (e) F.
    Although no characteristic neuropathological abnormality
    has yet been found in the brains of schizophrenic patients,
    there is growing consensus that temporal horns of the
    lateral ventricles are enlarged and abnormalities are
    prominent on the left side of the brain.

30. (a) T.
    (b) T.

(c) F.
(d) F. Shaping is a type of operant conditioning.
(e) F.

31. (a) F. It is usually reversible with withdrawal of the drug.
(b) T.
(c) T.
(d) T.
(e) F. Correlation is better with EEG, while there is poor correlation with serum levels.

32. (a) F.
(b) F.
(c) T.
(d) T.
(e) T.
Gestalt theory was developed in Germany under the influence of 7 men, including Max Westheimer and Kurt Lewin. In terms of motivation, the patients learn to recognize their needs at any given time and how the drive to satisfy those needs may influence their current behaviour.

33. (a) F. Insula, also known as the Island of Reil, is an area of the cerebral cortex.
(b) T.
(c) F. Diencephalon surrounds the third ventricle and is not a part of basal ganglia.
(d) T.
(e) T.

34. (a) T.
(b) T.
(c) F. The majority of cases are due to trisomy 21, a non-disjunction during meiosis.
(d) F. It is always irreversible in all cases.
(e) F. It is usually less than that of the general population.

35. (a) T.
(b) F.

(c) T.
(d) T.
(e) T.
GABA A receptors are linked to chloride channels and
GABA B channels are linked to calcium or potassium
channels.

36. (a) T.
     (b) F.
     (c) F.
     (d) T.
     (e) F.
Talcott Parsons' formulation of society's expectations
about the sick role involve 2 rights and 2 obligations: the
obligation to seek medical help and to define the state of
being sick as undesirable.

37. (a) T.
     (b) T.
     (c) T.
     (d) T.
     (e) F. The Mann-Whitney U test is essentially a test of
              significance.

38. (a) T.
     (b) T.
     (c) F.
     (d) T.
     (e) T.
Ethology has contributed to the understanding of human
behaviour and also emphasized particular avenues of
therapeutic approach in psychiatric care.

39. (a) T.
     (b) T.
     (c) T.
     (d) T.
     (e) T.
All these instruments measure different types of
phenomenology; e.g. Feighner Criteria are used for
diagnosis of depression.

40. (a) T.
    (b) T.
    (c) T.
    (d) F. Chloride channels are implicated in the mechanism
             of actions of anxiolytic drugs.
    (e) T.

41. (a) T.
    (b) F.
    (c) T.
    (d) T.
    (e) F.

42. (a) T. Such a reaction is produced by stimulation of the
             limbic system.
    (b) F. Anterior nucleus of the thalamus is part of the
             limbic system.
    (c) T.
    (d) T.
    (e) F. The globus pallidus is a part of the basal ganglia.

43. (a) T.
    (b) T.
    (c) F. Double-blind refers to the design of the study
             where both the observer and patient are unaware of
             the independent variables when measuring the
             dependent variables.
    (d) T.
    (e) T.

44. (a) T. The whole is greater than the sum of its parts. Other
             principles include ground differentiation.
    (b) T.
    (c) F.
    (d) T.
    (e) T.

45. (a) T.
    (b) F.
    (c) F.
    (d) T.

(e) F

The calcium channels open in response to membrane depolarization. They are subdivided into a low-voltage activator and a high-voltage activator, which are further divided into 2 subtypes. The calcium channel blockers do not influence neurotransmitter release.

46. (a) F.
    (b) F.
    (c) T.
    (d) F.
    (e) F.

Interracial contact is the most powerful way of decreasing racial prejudice; the others do so but in a less effective manner.

47. (a) F. It is an associated feature in some patients.
    (b) T.
    (c) T.
    (d) T.
    (e) F. Patients have an increased incidence of umbilical hernias.

48. (a) T.
    (b) T.
    (c) T.
    (d) F.
    (e) T.

It is noticed that a significant placebo response in the first week or two occurs in antidepressant drug trials, but it is not necessarily true for other types of drug trials.

49. (a) F.
    (b) T.
    (c) F.
    (d) F.
    (e) T.

There is no evidence for genetic predisposition. Although several hypotheses have been forwarded, including changes in receptor numbers and affinity, receptor sensitivity and levels of endogenous ligands, no hypothesis satisfactorily explains the mechanism of persistent withdrawal. Two personality types have been consistently identified: (i) Those who show impulsiveness and intolerance to intense emotion; (ii) those with dependent and avoidant personalities.

50. (a) F.
    (b) T.
    (c) F.
    (d) F.
    (e) T.
Variable ratio is the hardest to extinguish, which is why gambling is difficult to treat. Fixed ratio reinforcement schedule involves reinforcing – e.g. 1 in 3 correct responses – and involves reinforcing after a fixed interval of time of continuous response. Primary reinforcement takes place through decrease of basic drives.

1. (a) T.
   (b) T.
   (c) T. Oligodendrocytes form the myelin sheaths of the central neurones, while the Schwann cells form the myelin of the peripheral neurones.
   (d) F.
   (e) T.

2. (a) F. The establishment of a cause-and-effect relationship requires a different procedure.
   (b) T.
   (c) T.
   (d) F. Different procedures are required to establish validity and reliability.
   (e) T.

3. (a) T.
   (b) F. An autosomal recessive disorder of protein metabolism.
   (c) F. An autosomal recessive disorder of lipid metabolism.
   (d) T.
   (e) T.

4. (a) T.
   (b) F. It is related to fixation at the anal phase.
   (c) T.
   (d) T.
   (e) F. It was described by Erik Erikson as a defect due to a failure to resolve adolescent issues.

5. (a) T.
   (b) T.
   (c) T.
   (d) F. It is more often found in neurotic patients.
   (e) T.

6. (a) F. It is a manifestation of attachment between infant
          and mother.
   (b) T. It usually takes place between the ages of 3 and 6
          years.
   (c) T. It usually takes place between the ages of 6 and 12
          years.
   (d) F. It is the second stage of cognitive development of
          the child, as proposed by Piaget.
   (e) T. It occurs between the ages of 12 and 18 years.

7. (a) T.
   (b) F. Stria terminalis is not considered a part of the limbic
          system.
   (c) T.
   (d) T.
   (e) T.

8. (a) T. One extra X-chromosome and 1 Barr body.
   (b) T. One extra Y-chromosome and no Barr body.
   (c) F. It is an autosomal recessive disorder of copper
          metabolism.
   (d) F. It is an autosomal recessive disorder of protein
          metabolism.
   (e) F. It is an autosomal trisomy 18.

9. (a) F.
   (b) F.
   (c) T.
   (d) T.
   (e) F.
   The tangles are paired helical filaments. The plaques consist
   of amyloid precursor protein deposits surrounded by
   astrocytic and microglial cells. Amyloid deposition occurs
   in blood vessels.

10. (a) T.
    (b) T.
    (c) F.
    (d) F.
    (e) T.
    Drive-reduction theory suggests that most people avoid
    extreme tension-producing situations, but that some seek
    out such situations. Biological and physiological
    homeostasis are a type of intrinsic theory of motivation.

11. (a) F.
    (b) F.
    (c) F.
    (d) T.
    (e) T.
    The Standard Error is a measure of how much variation in
    test results is due to chance and error and how much is due
    to experimental influences.

12. (a) T.
    (b) T.
    (c) T.
    (d) T.
    (e) T.

13. (a) T.
    (b) F. The concrete operational stage is associated with the
        mastery of conservation.
    (c) T.
    (d) F. The formal operational stage is associated with
        detaching logic from immediate experience.
    (e) T.

14. (a) T. Fragile X syndrome and Lesch-Nyhan syndromes
        are X-linked recessive disorders.
    (b) T.
    (c) F. X-linked dominant disorder.
    (d) F. It is thought not to follow Mendelian inheritance.
    (e) F. It is due to an autosomal abnormality in the form of
        trisomy 13.

15. (a) T.
    (b) F.
    (c) F.
    (d) F.
    (e) T.

16. (a) T.
    (b) F.
    (c) T.
    (d) F.
    (e) T.
    Answer (b) refers to a reverse agonist, and answer (d) refers to an antagonist.

17. (a) T.
    (b) F.
    (c) T.
    (d) F.
    (e) T.
    Maslow's unified theory describes a hierarchy of needs ranked according to survival importance. It includes physical safety and self-actualization.

18. (a) F.
    (b) F. Adolescent turmoil used to be considered inevitable and beneficial. It probably arises due to stress in dealing with the various developmental tasks of adolescence.
    (c) F.
    (d) T.
    (e) T.

19. (a) F. A defect of iduronate sulphatase.
    (b) F. A defect of copper metabolism.
    (c) T. A defect of hexosa-minidase A.
    (d) T. A defect of galacto-cerebroside.
    (e) F. A defect of spingomyelinase.

20. (a) T.
    (b) T.

    (c) T. White matter changes as seen on MRI also occur
          away from the ventricles and in post-mortem
          studies. These lesions correspond to multiple
          sclerosis plaques.
    (d) T.
    (e) T.

21. (a) T.
    (b) T.
    (c) T.
    (d) F. They measure values other than central tendency.
    (e) F.

22. (a) F.
    (b) F.
    (c) F.
    (d) T.
    (e) T.

23. (a) T.
    (b) F.
    (c) F.
    (d) F.
    (e) F.
The PSE provides criteria for severity as well, since it
assesses the patient's mental state at the interview and in the
previous month; information about past illnesses is not
obtained. The SADS is a widely used interview schedule in
the USA. It covers a wide range of conditions, including
personality disorders and alcohol-related syndrome, unlike
the PSE.

24. (a) F.
    (b) F.
    (c) T.
    (d) T.
    (e) F. $P > 0.001$ indicates a highly statistically significant
          association.

25. (a) F.
    (b) F.
    (c) F.
    (d) F.
    (e) T.
    Nausea, vomiting, sedation, antidystonic reactions and
    tardive dyskinesia are due to blockade of dopaminergic
    neurotransmission.

26. (a) T.
    (b) F.
    (c) F.
    (d) T.
    (e) F.
    Identification is used by adolescents. Inhibition,
    intellectualization and isolation are neurotic defence
    mechanisms seen in adults under stress.

27. (a) F.
    (b) T.
    (c) T.
    (d) T.
    (e) F.

28. (a) F. Droperidol is a butyrophenone.
    (b) T.
    (c) F. Clozapine is a dibenzodiazepine. Loxapine is a
           dibenzoxazepine.
    (d) T.
    (e) F. Risperidone is a benzisoxazole.

29. (a) F.
    (b) F.
    (c) T.
    (d) T.
    (e) T.
    The Thurstone scale is where the subject is presented with a
    range of statements in which the subject ticks those he or
    she agrees with. In the Likert scale the subject is presented
    with a number of statements with which he or she indicates
    agreement on a 5-point scale.

30. (a) T.
    (b) T.
    (c) T.
    (d) T.
    (e) T.

31. (a) F. The consent of patient's next of kin is not legally
            valid.
    (b) T. The provisions of consent to treatment require the
            patient's informed consent under voluntary status.
    (c) F.
    (d) T.
    (e) T.

32. (a) T. The optic nerve is the sensory nerve of the retina.
            The optic chiasma is situated medial to the internal
            carotid arteries.
    (b) F.
    (c) F.
    (d) T.
    (e) T.

33. (a) T.
    (b) T.
    (c) T.
    (d) T.
    (e) F. They cause depolarization of neurones.

34. (a) T. It is a bimodal type of distribution.
    (b) T.
    (c) T.
    (d) F. In fact, it requires events to be independent.
    (e) T.

35. (a) F.
    (b) T.
    (c) F.
    (d) T.
    (e) F.
    Idiographic theories are concerned with individual

uniqueness and based on the study of the individual. Nomothetic theories are concerned with personality structure, and are based on studies of populations. Eysenck (type theory) and Cattell (trait theory) proposed nomothetic theories.

36. (a) F.
    (b) F.
    (c) T.
    (d) T.
    (e) T.
The primary energy source to the brain is glucose. Unlike other tissues, the brain cannot utilize lipids and proteins for energy. The brain has little glycogen storage. It can utilize some of the ketone bodies when their level is high.

37. (a) T. Commonly observed symptoms but not necessarily true withdrawal symptoms.
    (b) F.
    (c) F.
    (d) T.
    (e) T.

38. (a) T.
    (b) F. They can be retrospective as well.
    (c) T.
    (d) T.
    (e) T.

39. (a) T.
    (b) T.
    (c) T.
    (d) F.
    (e) T.
Ethnic bonds appear to be learned rather than biologically determined. The fixed action pattern is a genetically established sequence of motor activity that is triggered by a sign stimulus to release that pattern of behaviour.

40. (a) T.
    (b) T.
    (c) F. Fluid intake restriction may lead to neurotoxicity.
    (d) T.
    (e) F. No specific EEG changes; however, they consist of increasing episodes of intermittent, high-amplitude, diffuse delta waves.

41. (a) T. 80% of growth hormone is secreted during slow-wave sleep.
    (b) F.
    (c) T.
    (d) T.
    (e) T.

42. (a) F.
    (b) T.
    (c) F.
    (d) F.
    (e) T.

43. (a) F. D1 receptors are coupled to adenylate cyclase, and they are not found in the pituitary gland.
    (b) T.
    (c) T.
    (d) T.
    (e) F.

44. (a) F.
    (b) F.
    (c) T.
    (d) T.
    (e) F.
    Maguire & Rutter (1976) found that final year medical students were seriously deficient in psychiatric interviewing techniques. Personal areas of the history were avoided, and if the patient volunteered these topics the student would shift the interview to more neutral topics.

45. (a) F. The infant demonstrates general hypotonia.
    (b) F. A large, protruding tongue is a common feature.
    (c) T.
    (d) T.
    (e) T.

46. (a) F.
    (b) F.
    (c) T.
    (d) F.
    (e) T.
    The blood–brain barrier separates the brain and
    cerebrospinal fluid from the blood. It is represented
    structurally by the capillary endothelium of the brain, the
    subarachnoid space and the arachnoid membrane. The cells
    are tightly bound together. The lipid-soluble substances
    pass readily into the brain, as opposed to proteins, which
    enter more slowly.

47. (a) T.
    (b) T.
    (c) T.
    (d) F.
    (e) T.
    According to Festinger's theory of cognitive dissonance,
    the more important the cognitions the more powerful the
    dissonance.

48. (a) T.
    (b) T.
    (c) T.
    (d) F.
    (e) T.
    Type A personality tends to have an increased rate of
    myocardial infarction and angina pectoris.

49. (a) T. Anterograde amnesia is particularly associated with
           high potency drugs.

(b) T.
(c) T.
(d) T. Maculopapular rashes are a rare allergic reaction.
(e) T.

50. (a) T.
    (b) F. The occlusion of anterior cerebral artery results in
          contralateral hemiparesis, affecting the lower limb
          more than the upper limb.
    (c) T.
    (d) T.
    (e) T.

Reference

Maguire, G. P. and Rutter, D. R. (1976) 'History taking for medical students. I. Deficiencies in performance. *Lancet* ii (7985), 556–58.

CLINICAL PSYCHIATRY
PAPER 1

1. *In acute depersonalization syndrome:*
   (a) There is an alteration in tactile perception.
   (b) Delusional perception is a common experience.
   (c) Perception of time is significantly altered.
   (d) Anxiety is no longer experienced.
   (e) Hyperventilation is a common feature.

2. *The recognized features of obsessional personality include:*
   (a) A persistent difficulty in establishing a sexual relationship.
   (b) Magical undoing.
   (c) Fear of dirt.
   (d) Projection.
   (e) Preoccupation with cleanliness.

3. *The characteristic features of schizophrenic thought disorders include:*
   (a) Perseveration.
   (b) Derailment.
   (c) Symbolization.
   (d) Neologism.
   (e) Thought echo.

4. *The dysmnesic syndrome of recent origin may result from:*
   (a) Carbon dioxide poisoning.
   (b) Carbon monoxide poisoning.
   (c) Ingestion of amphetamines.
   (d) Nicotinic acid deficiency.
   (e) Ingestion of lysergic acid diethylamide (LSD).

5. *The following statements about suicide are correct:*
   (a) There is a history of attempted suicide in about 40% of cases.
   (b) Successful suicide is most often preceded by an attempted suicide in the previous 3 months.
   (c) The current trend indicates a shift towards late middle age for the maximum risk of suicide.
   (d) Psychopathic personalities are more likely to commit suicide than the general population.
   (e) Marital status offers some protection against suicide.

6. *Persecutory delusions in the elderly:*
   (a) Occur in about 10% of those over 65 years of age.
   (b) Usually precede the onset of dementia.
   (c) May lead to long-term hospitalization.
   (d) Are usually accompanied by Schneider's First Rank symptoms.
   (e) Usually do not respond to conventional neuroleptic drugs.

7. *The following statements about self-inflicted harm in elderly people are correct:*
   (a) Men are more often involved than women.
   (b) It is often precipitated by financial stress.
   (c) It has lower mortality than in the younger age group.
   (d) It is often associated with a significant mental disorder.
   (e) Bereavement is considered an important precipitant.

8. *Pharmacological treatments are particularly useful in the following conditions:*
   (a) Gilles de la Tourette's syndrome.
   (b) Pica.
   (c) Fire setting.
   (d) School refusal.
   (e) Hyperkinetic syndrome.

9. *The majority of homosexuals:*
   (a) Are effeminate.
   (b) Are consistently active or passive partners in their relationships.

    (c) Have multiple relationships.
    (d) Have an identifiable chromosomal or endocrine disorder.
    (e) Have an above-average sex-drive.

10. *The recognized features of epileptic children include:*
    (a) Wide variation of concentration.
    (b) Nocturnal fits in the majority of children.
    (c) Below-average intelligence.
    (d) Deafness.
    (e) Déjà vu.

11. *In Alzheimer's disease:*
    (a) Vasodilators are effective in a significant proportion of cases.
    (b) About 40% of patients suffer from arteriosclerosis.
    (c) More females than males are affected.
    (d) Depression is often a first presenting symptom.
    (e) Involuntary movements of hands occur in a majority of cases.

12. *Facial pain:*
    (a) May be a variant of migraine.
    (b) Is an associated feature of bipolar affective disorder.
    (c) If it responds to carbamazepine, it is likely to be trigeminal neuralgia.
    (d) May respond to antidepressant drugs even in the absence of a depressed mood.
    (e) May respond to cognitive-behavioural methods.

13. *The characteristic features of supportive psychotherapy include the following:*
    (a) It is usually concerned with neurotic symptoms.
    (b) The emphasis is on problem solving and adaptation in the present.
    (c) It involves empathic listening and non-possessive warmth.
    (d) One of its major concerns is to maintain a positive therapist–patient relationship.
    (e) It requires continuous and consistent support of the family members.

14. *The diagnostic features of bulimia nervosa include:*
    (a) Fear of being unable to control eating.
    (b) Depressed mood.
    (c) Insecure sexual relationship.
    (d) Insignificant loss of weight.
    (e) Amenorrhoea.

15. *Biological changes seen in mania include:*
    (a) Increased platelet monoamine levels.
    (b) Increased serum cortisol levels.
    (c) Reduction in thyroid stimulating hormone response to thyroid releasing factor.
    (d) Increased glucose tolerance.
    (e) Diffuse abnormalities on EEG recording.

16. *The characteristic features of Kretschmer's sensitivity reaction include:*
    (a) Ideas of reference.
    (b) Auditory hallucinations.
    (c) Shameful inadequacy.
    (d) Ruminations about personal achievements.
    (e) Low threshold for blushing.

17. *Short-lived paranoid psychosis with auditory hallucinations is likely to be caused by use of:*
    (a) Barbiturates.
    (b) Procyclidine.
    (c) Cannabis.
    (d) Alcohol.
    (e) Lysergic acid diethylamide.

18. *The recognized features of agoraphobic syndrome include:*
    (a) Fear of overcrowded places.
    (b) Fear of going out alone.
    (c) Fear of staying indoors.
    (d) Fear of traffic.
    (e) Avoidance of public places.

19. *Repeated periods of clouded consciousness with intermittent lucid intervals are a recognized feature of:*
    (a) Creutzfeldt-Jacob disease.
    (b) Depressive stupor.
    (c) Subdural haemorrhage.
    (d) Subarachnoid haemorrhage.
    (e) Wernicke's encephalopathy.

20. *Homicidal behaviour exhibited by a patient suffering from a severe bipolar affective disorder:*
    (a) Is common during the depressed phase.
    (b) Is common during the manic phase.
    (c) Is very likely to be directed at the members of the family.
    (d) Is invariably followed by suicidal behaviour.
    (e) Represents an alternative to a suicidal attempt.

21. *Over-breathing can produce:*
    (a) Urinary incontinence.
    (b) Parasthesias in one hand.
    (c) Profuse salivation.
    (d) Carpopedal spasm.
    (e) Convulsions.

22. *The characteristic features of people who repeatedly attempt deliberate self-harm include:*
    (a) A background of disrupted family life.
    (b) Presence of a psychiatric disorder in the majority of people.
    (c) Long-term unemployment.
    (d) Residence in a middle-class suburban area.
    (e) Low intelligence.

23. *Biological families of patients suffering from schizophrenia show an increased prevalence of:*
    (a) Organic disorders.
    (b) Bipolar affective disorders.
    (c) Alcohol-related problems.
    (d) Alzheimer's disease.
    (e) Mental subnormality.

24. *Regular consumption of the following drugs may lead to physical dependence:*
    (a) Dipipanone.
    (b) Dihydrocodeine.
    (c) Orphenadrine.
    (d) Viloxazine.
    (e) Amitriptyline.

25. *The clear contra-indications for unilateral Electroconvulsive Therapy (ECT) include:*
    (a) Pregnancy in the first trimester.
    (b) Depressive stupor in a severely mentally handicapped patient.
    (c) Acute catatonic schizophrenia.
    (d) Raised intracranial pressure.
    (e) A recent cerebrovascular accident.

26. *The following statements about supportive psychotherapy are correct:*
    (a) It is based on the principles of collective unconsciousness.
    (b) It deals with the impact of chronic physical illness on the patient.
    (c) The therapist is active and directive.
    (d) It is not useful in chronic schizophrenic patients.
    (e) It involves cognitive restructuring, reassurance and reinforcement.

27. *The following statements about a 75-year-old man with severe depressive illness are correct:*
    (a) Hospital admission is essential for successful treatment.
    (b) He presents a significantly higher suicidal risk than a 20-year-old severely depressed man.
    (c) Electroconvulsive Therapy (ECT) should not be given if there is evidence of cognitive impairment.
    (d) Monoamine oxidase inhibitors are contra-indicated.
    (e) He certainly has a shortened life expectancy.

28. *The characteristic features of psychopathic personality disorder include:*
    (a) Self-mutilation.
    (b) Repeated overdoses.
    (c) Loss of impulse control.
    (d) Guilt feelings about one's actions.
    (e) Homicidal tendencies.

29. *The recognized features of morbid jealousy include the following:*
    (a) It is commonly associated with alcohol abuse.
    (b) It is frequently associated with cocaine abuse.
    (c) It is commoner in women.
    (d) It is often associated with homicide.
    (e) It is rarely associated with schizophrenia.

30. *School refusal presenting for the first time in a 14-year-old boy:*
    (a) Is usually associated with antisocial behaviour.
    (b) Is often associated with depression.
    (c) Should be referred to social services rather than psychiatrists.
    (d) Would necessitate an immediate change of school.
    (e) Poses a significant risk of the development of agoraphobic symptoms in adulthood.

31. *In hysterical conversion syndrome the symptoms:*
    (a) Reduce conscious anxiety.
    (b) Occur in the hysterical personality.
    (c) Are mediated via the autonomic nervous system.
    (d) Are symbolic representations of intra-psychic conflicts.
    (e) Disappear as soon as the primary gain is achieved.

32. *The diagnostic features of depression include:*
    (a) Hyperamnesia.
    (b) Hyperphagia.
    (c) Impaired attention span.
    (d) Impaired short-term memory.
    (e) Reduced time spent in sleep.

33. *Microcephaly can occur because of:*
    (a) A recessive gene.
    (b) Smoking during the first 2 trimesters of pregnancy.
    (c) Rubella infection during the third trimester of pregnancy.
    (d) Toxaemia of pregnancy.
    (e) Exposure to X-ray radiation during pregnancy.

34. *The following statements about various legal provisions are correct:*
    (a) 'Testamentary capacity' means an ability to give evidence in a court of law.
    (b) The Court of Protection is empowered to give instructions as how to make a valid will.
    (c) Psychiatric patients cannot give evidence in the higher law courts.
    (d) 'Unfit to plead' results in an admission to a special hospital until fit to plead as decided by the Home Secretary.
    (e) 'Criminal responsibility' means that a child of 14 years and over is presumed to be fully responsible.

35. *Biological changes commonly seen in depression include:*
    (a) Increased thyroid-stimulating hormone response to thyroid-releasing factor.
    (b) Reduced cortisol suppression.
    (c) Increased prolactin level.
    (d) Decreased melatonin level.
    (e) Increased ACTH level.

36. *Absence seizures:*
    (a) Are a common cause of drop attacks.
    (b) Are diagnosed by 3-per-second spike and wave activity on an EEG.
    (c) Usually occur after puberty.
    (d) Respond best to carbamazepine.
    (e) Usually lead to development of generalized seizures in adult patients.

37. *The disorders of motor activity most commonly associated with schizophrenia include:*
   (a) Negativism.
   (b) Automatic obedience.
   (c) Perseveration.
   (d) Blepharo spasm.
   (e) Eyelid tremors.

38. *The following statements about ICD and DSM classification systems are correct:*
   (a) ICD10 specifies a minimum duration of 1 month for the diagnosis of depression.
   (b) DSMIIIR specifies a minimum of 2 months' duration for the diagnosis of schizophrenia.
   (c) ICD10 does not specify any time period for the diagnosis of schizophrenia.
   (d) ICD10 is an alpha-numeric coding system with a single letter followed by 2 numbers with a numeric subdivision.
   (e) DSMIIIR is a categorical diagnostic system with operationally defined criteria.

39. *The diagnostic features of Korsakoff's syndrome include:*
   (a) Lateral nystagmus.
   (b) Pseudologia fantastica.
   (c) Marked suggestibility.
   (d) Clouding of consciousness.
   (e) Auditory hallucinations.

40. *Urinary incontinence in the elderly can be reduced by:*
   (a) Promazine.
   (b) Special underclothes (e.g. Kanga pants).
   (c) Consideration of the design of the ward.
   (d) Supervision by the nurses.
   (e) Toilet training.

41. *Antimuscarinic (anticholinergic) drugs:*
   (a) Produce miosis.
   (b) Are known to produce visual hallucinations.
   (c) Are known to increase dyskinesia.

    (d) Reduce the plasma level of neuroleptic drugs.
    (e) Should not be prescribed simultaneously with neuroleptic drugs.

42. *Tactile hallucinations are recognized features in the following:*
    (a) Alcoholic polyneuropathy.
    (b) Cocaine abuse.
    (c) Anorexia nervosa.
    (d) Dermatitis artefecta.
    (e) Multiple sclerosis.

43. *The following statements about bipolar affective disorder are correct:*
    (a) Their incidence and prevalence are higher in males than females.
    (b) The onset of illness is earlier by 10–15 years compared with that of unipolar affective disorder.
    (c) There is a familial consistency in treatment responses in both sexes.
    (d) The incidence of depression in first-degree relatives is higher in bipolar affective disorder than in unipolar affective disorder.
    (e) The majority of patients suffering from this disorder recover fully after a course of lithium carbonate.

44. *The examination of eyes provides a diagnostic support in addition to clinical features in the following conditions:*
    (a) Glucose-6-phosphatase deficiency.
    (b) Wilson's disease.
    (c) Tay-Sachs' disease.
    (d) An overdose with barbiturates.
    (e) Colour blindness.

45. *Depression is a recognized presenting symptom of the following:*
    (a) Huntington's chorea.
    (b) Alzheimer's disease.
    (c) Schizophrenia.
    (d) Parkinson's disease.
    (e) Multiple disseminated sclerosis.

46. *Tricyclic antidepressant drugs:*
    (a) Produce cardiac failure due to negative inotropic effect on the myocardium.
    (b) Should not be given to patients with early cataracts.
    (c) Are known to produce depersonalization.
    (d) Invariably lead to fatal toxicity in an overdose.
    (e) Should not be combined with lithium carbonate.

47. *The complications of bulinia nervosa include:*
    (a) Erosion of dental enamel.
    (b) Parotid enlargement.
    (c) Epileptic seizures.
    (d) Menstrual disturbances.
    (e) Peptic ulcer.

48. *The following statements about bonding failure are correct:*
    (a) Biological depression in mother is an important factor.
    (b) Anakastic personality of the mother is an important factor.
    (c) 'Participative modelling' is a useful therapeutic approach.
    (d) Supportive psychotherapy is a useful therapeutic approach.
    (e) Abnormalities in the baby are of little significance in its aetiology.

49. *The clinical features of untreated cretinism include:*
    (a) Lethargy.
    (b) A large tongue.
    (c) Short stature.
    (d) Normal appearance at birth.
    (e) Hypotonia.

50. *Social class difference is found in:*
    (a) Childhood psychiatric disorder.
    (b) Suicide.
    (c) Obsessive compulsive disorder.
    (d) Anorexia nervosa.
    (e) Puerperal psychosis.

CLINICAL PSYCHIATRY
PAPER 2

1. *Depression is a recognized presenting feature of the following disorders:*
   (a) Pheochromocytoma.
   (b) Carcinoma of the pancreas.
   (c) Hypothyroidism.
   (d) Hyperparathyroidism.
   (e) Hyperthyroidism.

2. *The common features of chronic alcoholism include:*
   (a) Relief drinking.
   (b) Delirium tremens.
   (c) Alcoholic hallucinosis.
   (d) Peripheral neuropathy.
   (e) A narrowing of the drinking repertoire.

3. *The essential features of cerebral trypanosomiasis include:*
   (a) Anorexia.
   (b) Insomnia.
   (c) Somnolence.
   (d) Weight gain.
   (e) Elated mood.

4. *The following are known complications of chronic alcoholism:*
   (a) Hypertension.
   (b) Parkinson's disease.
   (c) Cerebellar ataxia.
   (d) Oesophageal varices.
   (e) Testicular atrophy.

5. *The clinical features of depersonalization syndrome include the following:*
   (a) It almost always precedes derealization.
   (b) It is considered to be a primary disturbance of ego functioning.
   (c) The person feels that the people around have changed.
   (d) Depressed mood.
   (e) Response to Electroconvulsive Therapy (ECT).

6. *The following statements about agoraphobic syndrome are correct:*
   (a) There is generalized anxiety in the majority of cases.
   (b) Clomipramine is an effective treatment.
   (c) Programme practice is a treatment of choice.
   (d) There is a higher incidence of sexual problems in a female group compared to a control population.
   (e) Most patients develop symptoms between ages 35 and 45 years.

7. *The following are associated with schizophreniform psychosis:*
   (a) Petit mal epilepsy.
   (b) Multiple sclerosis.
   (c) Hypothyroidism.
   (d) Parkinson's disease.
   (e) Diabetes mellitus.

8. *The factors significantly associated with repetition of deliberate self-harm include:*
   (a) Lower socioeconomic class.
   (b) Criminal behaviour.
   (c) Old age.
   (d) Male sex.
   (e) Early parental loss.

9. *Fugue states are known to occur in the following:*
   (a) Narcolepsy.
   (b) Depression.
   (c) Severe anxiety disorder.
   (d) Psychomotor epilepsy.
   (e) Hypoglycaemia.

10. *The characteristic features of systemic psychotherapy include:*
    (a) A focus on the symptomatic behaviour which occurs in a particular setting.
    (b) It is an interpersonal approach concentrating on dysfunctional relationship in a social group.
    (c) It involves regular analysis of transference and countertransference.
    (d) It is based on the principles of systematic desensitization.
    (e) It focuses primarily on the individual behaviour in question.

11. *The following are important in the aetiology of visual hallucinations in the elderly:*
    (a) Treatment with anticholinergic drugs.
    (b) Paraphrenia.
    (c) Severe visual impairment.
    (d) Untreated depression.
    (e) Treatment with antihypertensive drugs.

12. *The following statement(s) about termination of pregnancy is (are) correct:*
    (a) The upper limit for termination is 24 weeks of pregnancy.
    (b) It is illegal to perform it on a girl under 16 without her consent.
    (c) Parents' permission must be obtained in cases of girls under the age of 16.
    (d) It can only be performed if the patient's general practitioner agrees.
    (e) Two medical certificates are required: one of them must be from a doctor approved under the Mental Health Act.

13. *A 45-year-old man of a previously stable personality is likely to suffer from depression if:*
    (a) He attempted to murder his wife.
    (b) He attempted to murder a passer-by.
    (c) He was convicted for drunk and disorderly behaviour.

(d) He is disoriented in time and place.

(e) He was convicted for indecent exposure.

14. *Unilateral Electroconvulsive Therapy (ECT):*
    (a) Is contra-indicated in multi-infarct dementia.
    (b) Should be used as the treatment of choice in elderly depressed patients.
    (c) Is not contra-indicated in a depressed patient with a recent cerebrovascular accident.
    (d) Is the treatment of choice in late paraphrenia.
    (e) Is more effective in the treatment of depersonalization than bilateral Electroconvulsive Therapy.

15. *Attention span is characteristically found to be impaired in:*
    (a) Brain damage sustained following a road traffic accident.
    (b) Hyperkinetic syndrome.
    (c) Depression.
    (d) Social phobia.
    (e) Pick's disease.

16. *The prognosis in obsessive compulsive disorder:*
    (a) Is better for rituals than ruminations.
    (b) Is worse in untreated cases.
    (c) Depends on the type of antidepressant drug used.
    (d) Can be improved by using a combination of a selective serotonin re-uptake inhibitor and behaviour modification techniques.
    (e) Is worse in a patient with a family history of the same disorder.

17. *The following are more likely to occur in the biological families of patients suffering from schizophrenia and brought up by adoptive parents:*
    (a) High prevalence of inadequate personality.
    (b) Epilepsy.
    (c) First cousin marriages.
    (d) Organic psychosis.
    (e) High prevalence of alcohol abuse.

18. *The factors significantly associated with completed suicide after parasuicide in young people include:*
    (a) Female sex.
    (b) Social class V.
    (c) Personality disorder.
    (d) Broken relationship.
    (e) Substance misuse.

19. *The following may be primary aetiological factors in sexual difficulties in an otherwise stable marriage:*
    (a) Latent homosexuality.
    (b) Assortative mating.
    (c) Fear of pregnancy.
    (d) Hidden transvestism.
    (e) Post-natal depression.

20. *In analytic psychotherapy, the therapist must always consider:*
    (a) The role of the family members in the therapy.
    (b) The omissions and errors by the patient.
    (c) His or her emotional response to the patient's behaviour.
    (d) The sexual contents of the patient's behaviour.
    (e) The Oedipus complex.

21. *Auditory hallucinations in clear consciousness occur in the following:*
    (a) Atropine poisoning.
    (b) Amphetamine abuse.
    (c) Alcohol abuse.
    (d) Lead poisoning.
    (e) Alzheimer's disease.

22. *A 10-year-old autistic girl:*
    (a) Is likely to have an attachment to an imaginary friend.
    (b) May have fleeting gaze contact with the therapist.
    (c) Is likely to have a higher performance than verbal Intelligence Quotient (IQ).
    (d) Will only speak by echoing what is said.
    (e) Is likely to show manifestations of fragile X syndrome.

23. *The following statements about murder are correct:*
    (a) In about three-quarters of murder cases, the victims had known the murderer.
    (b) In about half of murder cases, the homicide suspects kill themselves.
    (c) The majority of murderers are mentally disordered.
    (d) It is unlawful killing without malice aforethought.
    (e) The higher courts have discretion in passing sentence, while the lower courts have no such privilege.

24. *The typical features of liver encephalopathy include:*
    (a) Hypersomnia.
    (b) Fast EEG activity.
    (c) Raised blood ammonia.
    (d) Impairment of consciousness.
    (e) Hyperkalaemia.

25. *The following statements about people who cross-dress are correct:*
    (a) They actively steal clothes from neighbours' washing lines.
    (b) They generally cross-dress in their own homes.
    (c) There is a confusion of gender identity.
    (d) Cross-dressing is an act which relieves inner tension.
    (e) They are homosexual in orientation.

26. *Recognized features of alcoholic hallucinosis include the following:*
    (a) The patient usually complains of seeing visions.
    (b) The patient is usually anxious and restless.
    (c) The consciousness is clouded.
    (d) Many of these patients have Schneider's First Rank symptoms.
    (e) They may occur at times of both relative increase and decrease in alcohol intake.

27. *The features typical of compensation neurosis include:*
    (a) Resolution of symptoms when the claim is settled.
    (b) Family history of the same disorder.
    (c) Frontal headaches.
    (d) Fainting attacks.
    (e) Severe difficulties with sleep.

28. *The therapeutic action of disulfiram in the treatment of alcoholism depends on:*
    (a) The fact that it diminishes craving for alcohol.
    (b) The principle of aversion therapy.
    (c) Its immediate metabolite, which reverses the sensitivity of the receptors for alcohol.
    (d) Fear of the potentially dangerous interaction with alcohol.
    (e) Its role as a deterrent to impulsive drinking.

29. *Excessive alcohol intake is associated with:*
    (a) Brain damage.
    (b) Old age.
    (c) Fatty liver.
    (d) Changes in peripheral synaptic transmission.
    (e) Cardiomyopathy.

30. *The frequently encountered clinical features of hyperventilation syndrome include:*
    (a) Tinnitus.
    (b) Carpopedal paraesthesias.
    (c) Substernal discomfort.
    (d) Syncope.
    (e) Nausea and vomiting.

31. *The prevalence of schizophrenia:*
    (a) Is higher in classes IV and V than in other classes.
    (b) Was higher in 1990 than 1890.
    (c) Is significantly lower in Ireland than England and Wales.
    (d) Is higher in monozygotic twins than dizygotic twins.
    (e) Is significantly higher in India than in the United Kingdom.

32. *The poor prognostic factors for anorexia nervosa include:*
    (a) Female gender.
    (b) Onset of illness in adolescence.
    (c) Bingeing.
    (d) Vomiting.
    (e) Parental conflict.

33. *The characteristic features of multi-infarct dementia include:*
    (a) Rapidly fluctuating course.
    (b) Severe loss of memory in the early stage.
    (c) Preponderance of women.
    (d) Parietal lobe dysfunction.
    (e) Reduced activity of choline acetyl transferase.

34. *The characteristic features of psychogenic amnesia include:*
    (a) Disturbance of recall.
    (b) Disturbance of retention.
    (c) Selective loss of memory about oneself.
    (d) Impairment of short-term memory.
    (e) Clouding of consciousness.

35. *Established causes of severe mental subnormality include:*
    (a) Hypertelorism.
    (b) Wilson's disease.
    (c) Fragile X syndrome.
    (d) XXY syndrome.
    (e) Sanfilippo's syndrome.

36. *Schneider's First Rank symptoms:*
    (a) Are pathognomic features of schizophrenia.
    (b) Are primary psychological symptoms from which all other symptoms are derived.
    (c) Occur in Alzheimer's disease.
    (d) Occur in bipolar affective disorder.
    (e) Are characteristic features of late paraphrenia.

37. *Kraepelin's 'mixed affective states' include:*
    (a) Delirious mania.
    (b) Excited depression.
    (c) Depressive stupor.
    (d) Schizo-affective psychosis.
    (e) Manic stupor.

38. *The complex visual hallucinations characteristically occur in:*
    (a) Multi-infarct dementia.
    (b) Parkinson's disease.

    (c) Temporal lobe lesions.
    (d) Occipital lobe lesions.
    (e) Atypical grief reaction.

39. *The following are pointers towards a psychiatric disorder in an 8-year-old child:*
    (a) Nail biting.
    (b) Thumb sucking.
    (c) Social withdrawal.
    (d) Nocturnal enuresis.
    (e) Consistent failure to attend school.

40. *The typical features of communicating hydrocephalus include:*
    (a) Papilloedema.
    (b) Neuronal loss in the cerebral cortex.
    (c) Urinary incontinence.
    (d) Bony lesions seen on skull X-ray.
    (e) Ataxia.

41. *The treatment plan of bulimia nervosa includes:*
    (a) Desensitization.
    (b) Imipramine.
    (c) Alprazolam.
    (d) Fluoxetine.
    (e) A behavioural contract.

42. *The following statements about culture-bound syndromes are correct:*
    (a) Latah is associated with homicidal attacks.
    (b) Anorexia nervosa is present in all societies.
    (c) Semen loss syndrome is a type of anxiety reaction.
    (d) Koro is caused by a virus infection.
    (e) Amok is found predominantly in Malaysia and South China.

43. *The characteristic features of lead poisoning include:*
    (a) Hypochromic anaemia.
    (b) Pica.
    (c) Diarrhoea.

(d) Wrist drop.

(e) Elevated free erythrocyte protoporphyrin.

44. *The characteristic features of Klinefelter's syndrome include:*
    (a) XXY chromosomes.
    (b) Gynaecomastia.
    (c) Testicular hypertrophy.
    (d) Severe learning disability in the majority of cases.
    (e) Cataract.

45. *The aetiological factors of failure of bonding include:*
    (a) A young mother.
    (b) An unwanted pregnancy.
    (c) The baby being nursed in a special care baby unit.
    (d) A complicated childbirth.
    (e) An absence of the father of the child.

46. *The following drugs are useful in depressed patients who have suffered from a recent myocardial infarction:*
    (a) Paroxetine.
    (b) Maprotiline.
    (c) Mianserin.
    (d) Doxepin.
    (e) Lofepramine.

47. *The outgoing mail of a compulsorily detained patient under the Mental Health Act cannot be intercepted if addressed to:*
    (a) The National Association of Mental Health.
    (b) The National Council for Civil Liberties.
    (c) The National Schizophrenia Fellowship.
    (d) The general practitioner.
    (e) The next of kin.

48. *The diagnostic features of XYY syndrome include:*
    (a) Above-average intelligence.
    (b) Above-average height for the general population.
    (c) Larger testicles.
    (d) Gynaecomastia.
    (e) Webbing of the neck.

49. *In psychoanalysis, resistance:*
    (a) Is an inevitable phenomenon.
    (b) Is a conscious unwillingness of the patient to continue in the therapy.
    (c) May be present even if the patient thinks he or she is cooperative.
    (d) Should be dealt with before starting the therapy.
    (e) Is a reaction to the countertransference of the therapist.

50. *Characteristic motor activity is observed in the following:*
    (a) Anorexia nervosa.
    (b) Premenstrual tension syndrome.
    (c) Alzheimer's disease.
    (d) Multiple sclerosis.
    (e) Down's syndrome.

CLINICAL PSYCHIATRY
PAPER 3

1. *The symptoms of acute schizophrenia can be exacerbated by giving the following agents:*
   (a) Endorphins.
   (b) L-Methionine.
   (c) Physostigmine.
   (d) Mescaline.
   (e) Phencyclidine.

2. *Amnesic confabulatory syndrome of longer than several weeks' duration is associated with:*
   (a) Nicotinic acid deficiency.
   (b) Gastric carcinoma.
   (c) Carbon monoxide poisoning.
   (d) Amphetamine poisoning.
   (e) Closed head injury.

3. *The correct statements about suicide include:*
   (a) Suicide rates are usually lower among Jews and Catholics than among Protestants.
   (b) The suicide rate in divorced people is about 4 times greater than that in married people.
   (c) Suicide is almost always preceded by an attempted suicide.
   (d) Suicide rates are usually higher in urban areas than in rural areas.
   (e) There is a past history of a depressive order in at least 50% of the victims.

4. *The following statement(s) about male homosexuality is (are) correct:*
   (a) About 10% of American males were exclusively homosexual in a study by Kinsey *et al.* (1948).

   (b) Homosexual behaviour is determined by hereditary factors.

   (c) Acts between men over 21 years of age with youths of 16 to 21 carry a penalty up to 10 years' imprisonment.

   (d) Acts with boys under 16 years of age carry penalties of up to life imprisonment.

   (e) Acts by youths aged 16 to 21 with anyone over 16 years can incur a penalty of up to 5 years' imprisonment.

5. *The following statement(s) about behaviour therapy for sexual dysfunction is (are) correct:*
   (a) The effect of the presence of both male and female therapists is greater than that of one therapist.
   (b) A ban on sole masturbation is usually necessary.
   (c) It involves banning sexual intercourse at the start in cases of premature ejaculation.
   (d) It involves patients keeping a diary of sexual activities.
   (e) It does not improve the prognosis of primary erectile impotence.

6. *The following names are paired with their associated concepts of schizophrenia:*
   (a) Morel – Dementia praecox.
   (b) Kraepelin – Demence precoce.
   (c) Bleuler – Autism.
   (d) Hecker – Catatonia.
   (e) Kahlbaum – Hebephrenia.

7. *A 60-year-old man of good premorbid personality exposes himself in a place for the first time. The following can be considered as a probable aetiological factor:*
   (a) Hypomania.
   (b) Erotomania.
   (c) Alzheimer's disease.
   (d) Silent myocardial infarction.
   (e) Generalized anxiety disorder.

8. *Vitamin B12 deficiency is known to cause:*
   (a) Depression.
   (b) Loss of ankle jerk.
   (c) Ocular palsy.
   (d) Limb paraesthesias.
   (e) Toxic confusional state.

9. *The characteristic features of sensitiver Beziehungswahn include:*
   (a) A sensitive delusion of reference.
   (b) An understandable psychological reaction.
   (c) Ideas of grandeur.
   (d) Delusional mood.
   (e) Thought echo.

10. *The characteristic features of alcoholic hallucinosis include:*
    (a) Clouding of consciousness.
    (b) Visual hallucinations.
    (c) Feeling of passivity.
    (d) Upward plantar reflex.
    (e) Derogatory auditory hallucinations.

11. *The following names are correctly paired with their psychological concepts of schizophrenia:*
    (a) Goldstein – Over-inclusive thought process.
    (b) Cameron – Concrete thinking.
    (c) Kelly – Construct theory.
    (d) Venables – Defective filter.
    (e) Broadbent – Over-arousal.

12. *The following drugs have a sedative effect in therapeutic dosages:*
    (a) Haloperidol.
    (b) Sulpiride.
    (c) Remoxipride.
    (d) Risperidone.
    (e) Clozapine.

13. *Acute intermittent porphyria is characteristically associated with:*
    (a) Skin sensitivity to ultraviolet light.
    (b) Aspirin compounds.
    (c) Persecutory delusions.
    (d) Clouding of consciousness.
    (e) Red urine.

14. *The following statements about social class are correct:*
    (a) It is decided by the Registrar General according to the occupation of the head of the family.
    (b) It is a reason for changing the incidence of Down's syndrome in Britain.
    (c) A definite relationship has been established between social class and suicide.
    (d) It accounts for increased incidence of schizophrenia among immigrants.
    (e) A definite relationship has been established between social class and depression.

15. *The ICD10 subcategories of schizophrenia include:*
    (a) Simple schizophrenia.
    (b) Latent schizophrenia.
    (c) Residual schizophrenia.
    (d) Post-schizophrenic depression.
    (e) Schizotypal disorder.

16. *The conditions which often show an improvement with intensive short-term psychoanalytic therapy include:*
    (a) Agoraphobia.
    (b) Dysmorphophobia.
    (c) Nosophobia.
    (d) Irritable bowel syndrome.
    (e) Transsexualism.

17. *The following statement(s) about depressed children is (are) correct:*
    (a) Fantasy is used to relieve it effectively.
    (b) A majority of untreated children become enuretic in adolescence.

(c) They may show social withdrawal.

(d) They usually fare less well in school.

(e) Most of them respond satisfactorily to selective serotonin re-uptake inhibitors.

18. *The following statement(s) about homosexuality is (are) correct:*
    (a) There is convincing evidence of abnormality of sex chromosomes.
    (b) The age for legal consent for homosexual intercourse is 18 years.
    (c) There is a significant deficiency of testosterone in a majority of cases.
    (d) There is convincing evidence of heredity determining homosexual behaviour.
    (e) Most homosexual women engage in heterosexual relationships at some time in their life.

19. *The following statement(s) about family therapy is (are) correct:*
    (a) The first step is to identify the context in which symptomatic behaviour occurs.
    (b) It aims at helping people to identify their problems in relation to others.
    (c) It may promote a re-organization of the whole system towards a healthier way of coping.
    (d) The whole family is not always required to be involved in the therapy.
    (e) It seeks to stimulate self-help potential of both the patient and key others.

20. *The names of the following people are associated with the development of the concept of psychopathy:*
    (a) Freud.
    (b) Asher.
    (c) Pinel.
    (d) Pritchard.
    (e) Kahn.

21. *The following drugs have a stimulating effect in therapeutic dosage in a majority of people:*
    (a) Lithium carbonate.
    (b) Fluoxetine.
    (c) Carbamazepine.
    (d) Moclobemide.
    (e) Citalopram.

22. *The risk of suicide is significantly associated with the following disorders:*
    (a) Obsessive compulsive disorder.
    (b) Anorexia nervosa.
    (c) Sociopathic personality disorder.
    (d) Huntington's chorea.
    (e) Social phobia.

23. *Schizophreniform psychosis may be associated more often than by chance with the following:*
    (a) Motor neurone disease.
    (b) Hypothyroidism.
    (c) Diabetes mellitus.
    (d) Parkinson's disease.
    (e) Multi-infarct dementia.

24. *Auditory hallucinations in clear consciousness characteristically occur in the following:*
    (a) Lead poisoning.
    (b) Alzheimer's disease.
    (c) Delirium tremens.
    (d) Cocaine abuse.
    (e) Mushroom poisoning.

25. *Persistent stealing from home by 6- to 10-year-old children is significantly associated with:*
    (a) Truancy.
    (b) A likelihood of antisocial personality as an adult.
    (c) Lack of guilt.
    (d) Less pocket-money than friends.
    (e) Depressive symptoms.

26. *The recognized features of anorexia nervosa include:*
    (a) Shoplifting of food.
    (b) Increased libido.
    (c) Decreased plasma TSH.
    (d) Decreased plasma cortisol.
    (e) Inversion of T wave on electrocardiograph.

27. *Specific reading retardation is significantly associated with:*
    (a) Low intelligence.
    (b) Speech delay.
    (c) Spelling difficulties.
    (d) Short-sightedness.
    (e) School refusal.

28. *The following drugs are absolutely contra-indicated in a patient with a recent history of myocardial infarction:*
    (a) Haloperidol.
    (b) Moclobemide.
    (c) Clozapine.
    (d) Fluvoxamine.
    (e) Lithium carbonate.

29. *A prisoner is not fit to plead if:*
    (a) He is admitted compulsorily to a psychiatric hospital under the Mental Health Act.
    (b) He does not understand the charge(s) or the significance of his plea.
    (c) He has not reached the age of 14 years.
    (d) He cannot understand the court procedures.
    (e) He experiences active psychotic symptoms.

30. *The recognized features of maternity blues include:*
    (a) A subjective 'confusion'.
    (b) Higher frequency among unmarried mothers.
    (c) A history of premenstrual tension.
    (d) Higher frequency among older mothers.
    (e) An antecedent of post-natal depression.

31. *The aims of group psychotherapy include:*
    (a) The improvement of interpersonal relations.
    (b) The conversion of groups into small democratic societies.
    (c) The achievement of significant changes in symptoms.
    (d) The achievement of limited adjustments in a disabling physical illness.
    (e) Provision of an opportunity to bring about substantial change in psychotic symptoms.

32. *The following are correct associations with reference to the concept/theory introduced:*
    (a) Berne – Paradoxical intention.
    (b) Maslow – Self-actualization.
    (c) Frankl – Transactional analysis.
    (d) Assagioli – Psychosynthesis.
    (e) Meyer – Psychobiology.

33. *The safe and satisfactory treatments of anorexia nervosa include:*
    (a) Individual psychotherapy.
    (b) Chlorpromazine.
    (c) Oral contraceptive drugs.
    (d) Amitriptyline.
    (e) Dynamic psychotherapy.

34. *The following condition(s) is (are) likely to accompany average intelligence in the majority of cases:*
    (a) Foetal rubella syndrome.
    (b) Neurofibromatosis.
    (c) Tuberous sclerosis.
    (d) Athetoid spastic paresis.
    (e) Spastic paraplegia.

35. *The essential features of pseudocyesis include:*
    (a) Abdominal distension.
    (b) Enlargement of uterus to the size of 12 weeks' pregnancy.
    (c) Quick resolution on diagnosis.
    (d) Fear of pregnancy.
    (e) Pigmentation of the breasts.

36. *The essential features of pathological grief reaction include:*
    (a) Searching behaviour by the bereaved person.
    (b) Visual hallucinations.
    (c) Auditory hallucinations.
    (d) Denial.
    (e) Resurrection of the deceased person's last illness.

37. *The indications for suitable subjects for group psychotherapy include:*
    (a) Persons who dominate other people.
    (b) Patients who have problems in relating to others.
    (c) Patients who are isolated with their problems.
    (d) Patients with a moderate degree of social anxiety.
    (e) Patients who are unable to establish long-lasting sexual relationships.

38. *The following are correct associations with reference to the concepts/therapy with which they are paired:*
    (a) Delay and Denicker – Chlorpromazine.
    (b) Pavlov – 'Basic anxiety'.
    (c) Griesinger – Unipolar psychosis.
    (d) K. Horney – Conditioned reflex.
    (e) Janet – Psychaesthenia.

39. *The term 'haptic hallucinations' refers to:*
    (a) Cutaneous perceptions of vague tingling.
    (b) Sensations of temperature change.
    (c) A feeling of movements just below the skin.
    (d) An experience of delusional perception.
    (e) A phenomenon of tingling and numbness over the abdomen.

40. *The diagnostic features of mania include:*
    (a) Paranoid delusion.
    (b) Disinhibition.
    (c) Over-spending of money.
    (d) Over-activity.
    (e) Transient depressed mood.

41. *The following drugs are absolutely contra-indicated in a patient with a recent history of myocardial infarction:*
    (a) Mianserin.
    (b) Imipramine.
    (c) Maprotiline.
    (d) Iprindole.
    (e) Sertraline.

42. *The symptoms of acute schizophrenia can be exacerbated by giving the following agents:*
    (a) L-Tryptophan.
    (b) 5-Hydroxytryptamine.
    (c) Dopamine.
    (d) Barbiturates.
    (e) Apomorphine.

43. *The names of the following people are associated with the history of hypnosis:*
    (a) Mesmer.
    (b) Braid.
    (c) Lièbault.
    (d) Breuer.
    (e) Coué.

44. *Severe memory impairment is characteristically caused by:*
    (a) Bilateral hippocampal damage.
    (b) Lesions in Broca's area.
    (c) Parietal lobe dysfunction.
    (d) Haemorrhages in mamillary bodies.
    (e) Damage to nucleus accumbens.

45. *The characteristic features of methyl alcohol poisoning include:*
    (a) Blindness.
    (b) Visual hallucinations.
    (c) Vomiting.
    (d) Severe occipital headaches.
    (e) Auditory hallucinations.

46. *The recognized reasons for increased incidence of delinquency include:*
    (a) Large family size.
    (b) Criminality in brother.
    (c) Low mean Intelligence Quotient (IQ).
    (d) Parental over-protection.
    (e) Low family income.

47. *The differential diagnoses of early infantile autism include:*
    (a) Over-dependency.
    (b) Aphasia.
    (c) Dyslexia.
    (d) Disintegrative psychosis.
    (e) Deafness.

48. *A 65-year-old woman is admitted to a psychiatric ward. She believes that she has cancer of the bowels in spite of evidence to the contrary. The diagnosis of a major depressive disorder is strongly suggested by:*
    (a) Late insomnia.
    (b) Worsening of the mood in the evening.
    (c) Loss of weight.
    (d) Psychomotor retardation.
    (e) Disorientation in time and place.

49. *Recognized indications for psychosurgery in the United Kingdom include:*
    (a) Intractable facial pain.
    (b) Intractable agoraphobia.
    (c) Chronic unremitting bipolar affective disorder.
    (d) Severe intractable generalized anxiety disorder.
    (e) Chronic unremitting obsessive compulsive disorder.

50. *In severe mental handicap:*
    (a) 80% of cases have a known cause.
    (b) Male-to-female ratio is 4 to 1.
    (c) Prenatal counselling significantly reduces its incidence.
    (d) 50% of cases are institutionalized.
    (e) Behaviour modification may improve behaviour in a majority of cases.

CLINICAL PSYCHIATRY
ANSWERS TO
PAPER 1

1. (a) F.
   (b) F.
   (c) T.
   (d) F.
   (e) F.
   Depersonalization syndrome is characterized by an unpleasant state of disturbed perception in which external objects or parts of the body are experienced as changed in various ways. It is associated with mild anxiety, depression and dejà vu. Two-thirds of the patients are women.

2. (a) F. A feature of psychopathic personality disorder.
   (b) F. A defence mechanism noticed in obsessive compulsive disorder.
   (c) F. A feature of obsessive compulsive disorder.
   (d) F. A defence mechanism not associated with obsessional personality.
   (e) T.

3. (a) F. Perseveration also observed in other conditions such as dementias and mental subnormality.
   (b) T.
   (c) F. Symbolization is one of the mechanisms of dream work.
   (d) T.
   (e) F.

4. (a) T.
   (b) T.
   (c) T.

(d) F. Nicotinic acid usually causes chronic dysmnesic syndrome.

(e) T.

5. (a) T. About two-thirds of patients who commit suicide have seen a health-care worker during the preceding three weeks.

(b) F.

(c) T.

(d) T. Psychopathic personalities kill themselves more often accidentally than with a deliberate intention.

(e) T.

6. (a) F. Persecutory delusions are part of late paraphrenia. Its prevalence rate is about 0.2 to 0.3%.

(b) F. Paranoid symptoms may precede the onset of dementia and usually respond to neuroleptic drugs.

(c) T.

(d) F.

(e) F.

7. (a) T. Unlike deliberate self-harm in young people, men are more likely to be involved. The mortality rate is higher than in the younger age group.

(b) F.

(c) F.

(d) T.

(e) T.

8. (a) T.

(b) F.

(c) F.

(d) F.

(e) T.

Behaviour modification is useful in pica, fire setting and school refusal.

9. (a) F.

(b) T.

(c) T.
(d) F. There is no convincing evidence of sex
        chromosomes or neuroendocrine system disorder.
(e) F.

10. (a) T.
    (b) F.
    (c) F.
    (d) F.
    (e) T.

11. (a) F.
    (b) F.
    (c) T.
    (d) T.
    (e) F.
Alzheimer's disease is of idiopathic origin which may have
a genetic basis in some patients. There is no evidence of
arteriosclerosis, as is the case with multi-infarct dementia.

12. (a) T.
    (b) F.
    (c) T.
    (d) T.
    (e) T.
Facial pain has many physical causes but it can be relieved
by antidepressant drugs, even though there is no evidence
of depression.

13. (a) T.
    (b) F.
    (c) F.
    (d) T.
    (e) F.
Supportive psychotherapy, a type of individual
psychotherapy, is used to help a person through a time-
limited crisis. The patient is encouraged to talk about his
problems.

14. (a) T.
    (b) F.
    (c) F.
    (d) T.
    (e) F.
    The other diagnostic features of bulimia include recurrent episodes of binge eating and persistent over-concern with body shape and weight. Depressed mood is common. Most patients are sexually active.

15. (a) T.
    (b) T.
    (c) T.
    (d) F.
    (e) F.
    In mania, glucose tolerance is unaffected and there are no EEG abnormalities.

16. (a) T.
    (b) F.
    (c) F.
    (d) F.
    (e) F.
    Kretschmer believed that 'sensitive' people develop suspicious ideas when faced with a deeply humiliating experience. Such ideas can easily be mistaken for persecutory delusions, i.e. sensitive delusions of reference (Sensitiver Beziehungswahn).

17. (a) F.
    (b) F.
    (c) T.
    (d) T.
    (e) T.

18. (a) T.
    (b) F.
    (c) F.
    (d) T.

(e) T.
Agoraphobic syndrome includes a fear of being in places or situations from which escape might be difficult.

19. (a) F. Creutzfeldt-Jacob disease is a progressive dementia. In depressive stupor, there is no impairment of consciousness.
    (b) F.
    (c) T.
    (d) F. In subarachnoid haemorrhage, there might be transient impairment of consciousness which might progress to coma.
    (e) T.

20. (a) F. Homicidal behaviour is not a common feature in either the depressed or the manic phase.
    (b) F.
    (c) T. It is not an alternative to a suicidal attempt but may be followed by one.
    (d) F.
    (e) F.

21. (a) F. Over-breathing can lead to urinary frequency, paraesthesias in limbs and dry mouth.
    (b) F.
    (c) F.
    (d) T.
    (e) T.

22. (a) T.
    (b) F.
    (c) T.
    (d) F.
    (e) F.
Such people are of average intelligence and come from a lower socioeconomic class. About 10 to 15% suffer from a detectable psychiatric disorder.

23. (a) F.
    (b) T.

    (c) T.
    (d) F.
    (e) F.

24. (a) T.
    (b) T.
    (c) F.
    (d) F.
    (e) F.

25. (a) F. But ECT is better avoided in the first trimester of
        pregnancy.
    (b) F.
    (c) F.
    (d) T.
    (e) T.

26. (a) F.
    (b) T.
    (c) T.
    (d) F.
    (e) T.
Supportive psychotherapy is based on the principles of
restoring or strengthening the defences and integrating
capacities that have been impaired. It uses the techniques
that help the patient feel more secure, accepted, protected,
encouraged and safe.

27. (a) T. ECT is probably the treatment of choice in elderly
        patients, but they can be successfully treated at
        home if adequate support is available.
    (b) T.
    (c) F.
    (d) F.
    (e) T.

28. (a) F.
    (b) F.
    (c) T.
    (d) F.

(e) F.
All other features are associated with psychopathic personality but are not considered characteristic of the disorder.

29. (a) F.
    (b) F.
    (c) F.
    (d) F.
    (e) F.
Morbid jealousy is associated with alcohol abuse in about 10% of cases. Male-to-female ratio is 2 to 1. It is noticed quite often in schizophrenia.

30. (a) F. An emotional disorder which needs to be treated by the psychiatric team.
    (b) T.
    (c) F.
    (d) F. It does not require a change of school.
    (e) T.

31. (a) F.
    (b) F.
    (c) F.
    (d) T.
    (e) F.
They reduce unconscious anxiety and only about 30% of patients have hysterical personality. The symptoms are mediated via the central nervous system.

32. (a) F.
    (b) F.
    (c) F.
    (d) F.
    (e) T.
All other symptoms except hyperamnesia occur in depression but are not necessarily diagnostic of depression.

33. (a) T.
    (b) F.

(c) F.
(d) F.
(e) T.

34. (a) F. 'Testamentary capacity' means an ability to make a valid will.
(b) F. The Court of Protection is empowered to look after the financial affairs of the patients.
(c) F. Psychiatric patients can give evidence in any court of law.
(d) T.
(e) T.

35. (a) F. Blunted release of TSH in response to TRF.
(b) T.
(c) F. Prolactin and ACTH levels appear to be unaffected in depression.
(d) T.
(e) F.

36. (a) F. There are brief disruptions of consciousness without convulsive movements.
(b) T.
(c) F. They usually begin in childhood between ages 5 and 7 and cease by puberty.
(d) F. The drugs of choice are sodium valproate and ethosuximide.
(e) F.

37. (a) T.
(b) T.
(c) F.
(d) F.
(e) F.
Perseveration is a disorder of speech. Blepharospasm and eyelid tremors may be idiopathic or iatrogenic in origin. They may be seen in schizophrenic patients.

38. (a) F. ICD10 requires a minimum duration of two weeks.
(b) F.

(c) F.
(d) T.
(e) T.
ICD10 requires a minimum duration of 2 weeks, while
DSMIIIR requires 1 week's duration of psychotic
symptoms.

39. (a) F. Such patients are often suggestible.
    (b) F.
    (c) F.
    (d) F.
    (e) F.

40. (a) T.
    (b) F.
    (c) T.
    (d) T.
    (e) T.

41. (a) F.
    (b) T.
    (c) T.
    (d) T.
    (e) T.

42. (a) F.
    (b) T.
    (c) F.
    (d) F.
    (e) F.

43. (a) T.
    (b) F. The mean age of onset of bipolar affective disorder
            is slightly older than that of unipolar affective
            disorder.
    (c) T.
    (d) F.
    (e) F.

44. (a) F.
    (b) T.
    (c) T.
    (d) T.
    (e) F.
    In Wilson's disease, golden brown, yellow or green corneal
    pigmentation known as Kayser-Fleischer ring, occurs,
    while in Tay-Sachs' disease a cherry-red macular spot, optic
    disc and retinal atrophy leads to blindness.

45. (a) T.
    (b) T.
    (c) T.
    (d) T.
    (e) T.

46. (a) T.
    (b) F. Tricyclic antidepressant drug can be used quite
        safely with lithium carbonate, and in patients with
        early cataract.
    (c) F.
    (d) F.
    (e) F.

47. (a) T.
    (b) T.
    (c) T.
    (d) T.
    (e) F.

48. (a) T.
    (b) T.
    (c) T.
    (d) T.
    (e) F. An abnormal baby may lead to its rejection by the
        mother.

49. (a) T.
    (b) T.
    (c) T.
    (d) T.
    (e) T.

50. (a) T.
    (b) T.
    (c) F.
    (d) T.
    (e) F.

CLINICAL PSYCHIATRY
ANSWERS TO
PAPER 2

1. (a) T.
   (b) T.
   (c) T.
   (d) T.
   (e) T.

2. (a) T.
   (b) F.
   (c) F.
   (d) F.
   (e) T.
   Delirium tremens is a withdrawal state. Peripheral
   neuropathy is a neurological complication. Alcoholic
   hallucinosis is an uncommon condition.

3. (a) T.
   (b) T.
   (c) T.
   (d) F. It is associated with weight loss and apathy.
   (e) F.

4. (a) F.
   (b) F.
   (c) T.
   (d) T.
   (e) T.

5. (a) F.
   (b) F.
   (c) F.
   (d) T.

(e) F.
Depersonalization syndrome is characterized by an unpleasant state of feeling unreal and experiencing an unreal quality to perceptions. On most occasions it is a secondary condition; treatment should be directed to the primary condition.

6. (a) T. Two peaks of onset: early or middle twenties and mid-thirties.
   (b) F.
   (c) T.
   (d) T.
   (e) F.

7. (a) F.
   (b) T.
   (c) T.
   (d) T.
   (e) F. Diabetes mellitus may be associated with depression, anxiety, cognitive impairment, restlessness and irritability.

8. (a) T.
   (b) T.
   (c) F.
   (d) F. Young females are most likely to repeat acts of deliberate self-harm.
   (e) F.

9. (a) F.
   (b) T.
   (c) T.
   (d) T.
   (e) T.

10. (a) T.
    (b) T.
    (c) F.
    (d) F.
    (e) T.

11. (a) T.
    (b) T.
    (c) F.
    (d) F.
    (e) F.

12. (a) T.
    (b) T.
    (c) F.
    (d) F.
    (e) F.

13. (a) T.
    (b) F.
    (c) T.
    (d) F.
    (e) T.
    In depression, aggression is usually directed towards
    oneself and close family, especially if suicide is
    contemplated.

14. (a) F. The contra-indications/indications for ECT are the
           same whether it is administered unilaterally or
           bilaterally.
    (b) T.
    (c) F.
    (d) F.
    (e) F.

15. (a) T.
    (b) T.
    (c) T.
    (d) F.
    (e) T.

16. (a) F. No difference in outcome between rituals and
           ruminations.
    (b) T.
    (c) F.
    (d) T.
    (e) F.

17. (a) T.
    (b) T.
    (c) F. First-cousin marriages are more likely to be
           associated with autosomal recessive disorders.
    (d) F.
    (e) T.

18. (a) F. Male sex is a significant factor.
    (b) T.
    (c) T.
    (d) F.
    (e) T.

19. (a) T.
    (b) F.
    (c) T.
    (d) T.
    (e) F.

20. (a) F. Family members are not involved in such therapy,
           however conflicts in relation to them are dealt
           with.
    (b) T.
    (c) T.
    (d) F.
    (e) F.

21. (a) F.
    (b) F.
    (c) T.
    (d) F.
    (e) T.

22. (a) T.
    (b) T.
    (c) T.
    (d) F.
    (e) F. Fragile X syndrome principally affects males and is
           the second most common cause of mental
           retardation after Down's syndrome.

23. (a) T.
    (b) F. Up to 30% of homicide suspects (especially women) kill themselves following murder.
    (c) F. About 50% of murderers are mentally abnormal and suffer from severe personality disorder, depression, schizophrenia or alcoholism.
    (d) F.
    (e) F.

24. (a) T.
    (b) F. The earliest EEG change is a slowing of the alpha rhythm and the appearance of 5–7 per second theta waves, which will replace alpha waves as consciousness is progressively impaired. Later, characteristic triphasic waves are seen, suggesting a poor prognosis.
    (c) T.
    (d) T.
    (e) F.

25. (a) F.
    (b) T.
    (c) T.
    (d) T.
    (e) F.

26. (a) F. It is characterized by auditory hallucinations, usually voices uttering insults or threats in clear consciousness.
    (b) T.
    (c) F.
    (d) F.
    (e) T.

27. (a) F. Compensation neurosis is a term used for psychologically determined physical or mental symptoms occurring when there is an unsettled claim for compensation. In some patients, the symptoms may persist for several years after compensation.

(b) F.
(c) T.
(d) T.
(e) F.

28. (a) F. Disulfiram acts by blocking the oxidation of alcohol so that acetaldehyde accumulates, which produces an unpleasant experience.
    (b) T.
    (c) F.
    (d) T.
    (e) T.

29. (a) T.
    (b) F.
    (c) T.
    (d) F.
    (e) T.

30. (a) F.
    (b) T.
    (c) T.
    (d) T.
    (e) F.
    The symptoms are due to cerebral vasoconstriction and respiratory acidosis.

31. (a) T.
    (b) F. There is no evidence that the prevalence was higher or lower in 1990 than in 1890.
    (c) F. High prevalence has been reported in Ireland.
    (d) T.
    (e) F. It has been reported as less in India than in the UK as the prognosis is better in the former country.

32. (a) F.
    (b) T.
    (c) F.
    (d) F.
    (e) F.

The only established factor predictive of outcome is the length of illness at presentation. It is also evident that an onset of illness in adolescence and male sex suggest a poor prognosis.

33. (a) F.
    (b) F.
    (c) F.
    (d) F.
    (e) F.
It is slightly more common in men than in women. Emotional and personality changes may appear first, followed by impairments of memory and intellect which fluctuate, but not rapidly. There is association between cognitive impairment and levels of choline acetyl transferase.

34. (a) T.
    (b) F.
    (c) T.
    (d) T.
    (e) T.
It usually begins abruptly. Some patients report a slight clouding of consciousness during the period immediately preceding the amnesia. The capacity to learn new information is retained in these patients.

35. (a) T.
    (b) F.
    (c) T.
    (d) F.
    (e) T.

36. (a) F. The presence of Schneider's First Rank symptoms in clear consciousness suggest schizophrenia, but their absence does not rule it out.
    (b) F.
    (c) F.
    (d) T.
    (e) T.

37. (a) F.
    (b) T.
    (c) F.
    (d) F.
    (e) T.

38. (a) F.
    (b) F.
    (c) T.
    (d) T.
    (e) F.

39. (a) F.
    (b) F.
    (c) T.
    (d) T.
    (e) T.
    Nail biting and thumb sucking are considered neurotic traits which have little relevance in psychiatric practice.

40. (a) F.
    (b) F.
    (c) T.
    (d) F.
    (e) T.

41. (a) T.
    (b) T.
    (c) F.
    (d) T.
    (e) T.
    Some antidepressant drugs like desipramine, trazodone and monoamine oxidase inhibitors also appear promising.

42. (a) F. Latah, found among Malaysian women, usually begins after a sudden frightening experience. The patient shows echolalia and echoproxia and is abnormally compliant in other ways.
    (b) T.
    (c) T.

(d) F. Koro is a psychogenic disorder, a type of acute anxiety reaction in which the patient fears that his penis is shrinking and may disappear into his abdomen and that he may die.

(e) T.

43. (a) T.
   (b) F. Pica is one of the main causes of lead toxicity; the other features include colicky abdominal pain, constipation, headache and irritability. Coma and convulsions occur in severe cases.
   (c) F.
   (d) T.
   (e) T.

44. (a) T.
   (b) T.
   (c) F.
   (d) F.
   (e) F.

The other characteristic features of Klinefelter's syndrome include hypogonadism, reduced or absent post-pubertal facial hair, a female distribution of pubic hair. Mild learning disability may occur, but many patients have an IQ in the normal range.

45. (a) F.
   (b) T.
   (c) T.
   (d) T.
   (e) F.

46. (a) T.
   (b) F.
   (c) T.
   (d) T. Use with caution with recent myocardial infarction.
   (e) F.

47. (a) F.
   (b) F.

(c) F.
(d) F.
(e) F.
Outgoing mail of a detained patient to his solicitors,
Member of Parliament, hospital managers, responsible
medical officer cannot be intercepted.

48. (a) F. Below-average intelligence.
 (b) T.
 (c) F. Testicles of normal size.
 (d) F. A feature of XXY syndrome (Klinefelter's).
 (e) F. A feature of XO (Turner's) syndrome.

49. (a) T.
 (b) F. Resistance is an unconscious interference in therapy
 which is dealt with as the therapy progresses.
 (c) T.
 (d) F.
 (e) F.

50. (a) T.
 (b) F.
 (c) T.
 (d) F.
 (e) F.

CLINICAL PSYCHIATRY
ANSWERS TO
PAPER 3

1. (a) F.
   (b) F.
   (c) F.
   (d) T.
   (e) T.
   Mescaline and phencyclidine are hallucinogens.

2. (a) T. Untreated nicotinic acid deficiency may lead to a
        state like Korsakoff's syndrome or to slowly
        progressing dementia.
   (b) T.
   (c) T.
   (d) F.
   (e) T.

3. (a) T.
   (b) F. Suicide rates are lowest among the married and are
        considered higher among the divorced, but certainly
        not 4 times higher.
   (c) F.
   (d) T.
   (e) T.

4. (a) T.
   (b) T.
   (c) F.
   (d) T.
   (e) F.
   Homosexual acts by men over 18 years of age with men
   aged 16–18 carry a penalty up to 5 years' imprisonment,
   and acts with boys under 16 carry a penalty of up to 10
   years' imprisonment.

5. (a) T.
   (b) T. It improves the prognosis of primary erectile impotence but to a limited extent.
   (c) T.
   (d) T.
   (e) F.

6. (a) F.
   (b) F.
   (c) T.
   (d) F.
   (e) F.
   Morel is associated with demence praecox, Kraepelin with dementia praecox, Hecker with hebephrenia and Kahlbaum with catatonia. Bleuler coined the term 'schizophrenia', and described the 4 As: autism, ambivalence, loosening of associations and flattening of affect.

7. (a) T.
   (b) F.
   (c) T.
   (d) T. Silent myocardial infarction may cause toxic confusional state, which in turn may tend to antisocial behaviour.
   (e) F.

8. (a) T. The hallmark of vitamin B12 deficiency is megaloblastic anaemia and its sequelae, like glossitis.
   (b) F.
   (c) F.
   (d) T. It also produces a complex neurologic syndrome of paraesthesias, posterior column features, etc.
   (e) T. It may occur in advanced cases.

9. (a) T.
   (b) T.
   (c) F.
   (d) F.

(e) F.
Kretschmer stressed the importance of the underlying personality in development of a delusion. As a sequel to a key experience, a delusion develops from sensitive ideas of reference, i.e. sensitiver Beziehungswahn.

10. (a) F.
    (b) F.
    (c) F.
    (d) F.
    (e) T.

11. (a) F. Goldstein is associated with concrete thinking and Cameron with over-inclusive thinking.
    (b) F.
    (c) T.
    (d) F.
    (e) F.
Venables is associated with over-arousal and Broadbent with defective filter theory.

12. (a) T.
    (b) F.
    (c) F.
    (d) F.
    (e) T.

13. (a) F. It is characterized by intermittent abdominal pain, peripheral neuropathy seizures, psychosis and basal ganglion abnormalities.
    (b) F.
    (c) F. Attacks are precipitated by numerous factors, including sulphonamides and barbiturates. Freshly voided urine is of normal colour but may turn dark on standing in light and air.
    (d) F.
    (e) F.

14. (a) T.
    (b) T.
    (c) F. Suicide rates are higher in social classes V and I than
        in the other social classes.
    (d) F. The incidence of schizophrenia is equal in all social
        classes.
    (e) F.

15. (a) T.
    (b) F.
    (c) T.
    (d) T.
    (e) F.
    ICD10 classifies schizophrenia (Code F20) as simple,
    hebephrenic, catatonic, undifferentiated, post-
    schizophrenic depression, and of residual type. Schizotypal
    disorder is a separate diagnostic category (Code F21).

16. (a) F.
    (b) F.
    (c) F.
    (d) F.
    (e) F.

17. (a) F.
    (b) F.
    (c) T.
    (d) T.
    (e) F. No systematic clinical studies of antidepressant
        drugs are available to date.

18. (a) F.
    (b) T.
    (c) F.
    (d) F. There is some evidence that homosexual behaviour
        is determined by heredity but it is not convincing.
        There is also no convincing evidence of abnormality
        in sex chromosomes or the neuroendocrine system.
    (e) T.

19. (a) T.
    (b) T.
    (c) T.
    (d) T.
    (e) T.

20. (a) F.
    (b) F.
    (c) T.
    (d) T.
    (e) F.
    The names of Freud, Asher and Kahn are associated with psychoanalysis, Munchausen's syndrome and anankastic personality, respectively.

21. (a) F.
    (b) T.
    (c) F.
    (d) T.
    (e) T.

22. (a) F.
    (b) T.
    (c) T.
    (d) T.
    (e) F.

23. (a) F.
    (b) T.
    (c) F.
    (d) T.
    (e) T.

24. (a) T.
    (b) T.
    (c) F. In delirium tremens, the hallucinations are associated with clouded consciousness.
    (d) T.
    (e) T.

25. (a) T.
    (b) T.
    (c) T.
    (d) F.
    (e) F.
Persistent stealing is a type of conduct disorder which is not significantly associated with items (d) and (e).

26. (a) T.
    (b) F.
    (c) T.
    (d) F. Plasma cortisol is increased and its normal diurnal variation lost. There is a marked reduction in libido at the onset of illness.
    (e) T.

27. (a) F. It is associated with impaired writing and spelling and average or above-average intelligence.
    (b) T.
    (c) T.
    (d) F.
    (e) F.

28. (a) T.
    (b) T.
    (c) F.
    (d) F.
    (e) T.

29. (a) F.
    (b) T.
    (c) F. The legal criteria of unfitness to plead do not include age and compulsory hospital admission.
    (d) T.
    (e) F.

30. (a) T.
    (b) F.
    (c) T.
    (d) F.

(e) F.
Maternity blues are more frequent among primigravida.
They are not related to marital status or age of the mother.
They are certainly not an antecedent of post-natal
depression, as it is a self-limiting condition lasting for a few
days.

31. (a) T.
    (b) F.
    (c) T.
    (d) T.
    (e) F.

32. (a) F.
    (b) T.
    (c) F.
    (d) T.
    (e) T.
The names of Berne and Frankl are associated with
transactional analysis and paradoxical intention,
respectively.

33. (a) T.
    (b) T.
    (c) F.
    (d) F.
    (e) F.

34. (a) F.
    (b) T.
    (c) F.
    (d) F.
    (e) T.

35. (a) T.
    (b) F.
    (c) T.
    (d) T.
    (e) T.
Psendocyesis is the occurrence of a false pregnancy with

amenorrhoea, abdominal distension (not necessarily enlargement of the uterus) and other changes similar to those of early pregnancy.

36. (a) T.
    (b) F.
    (c) F.
    (d) F.
    (e) T.
Other features include: phobic avoidance of persons, places or things related to the deceased; a total lack of grieving, with anger directed towards others; and over-idealization of the deceased.

37. (a) F.
    (b) T.
    (c) F. Such people do not benefit from group psychotherapy.
    (d) T.
    (e) T.

38. (a) T.
    (b) F.
    (c) F.
    (d) F.
    (e) T.
The names of Pavlov, Griesinger and K. Horney are associated with classical conditioning, unitary psychosis and 'basic anxiety', respectively.

39. (a) T.
    (b) F.
    (c) T.
    (d) F.
    (e) F.

40. (a) F.
    (b) T.
    (c) T.
    (d) T.
    (e) T.

41. (a) F.
    (b) T.
    (c) T.
    (d) T.
    (e) F.

42. (a) F.
    (b) F.
    (c) T.
    (d) F.
    (e) F.

43. (a) T.
    (b) T.
    (c) T.
    (d) T.
    (e) T.

44. (a) T.
    (b) F.
    (c) F.
    (d) T.
    (e) F.

45. (a) T.
    (b) F.
    (c) T.
    (d) F.
    (e) F.
    The other features include metabolic acidosis, tachypnea,
    confusion, convulsions and coma.

46. (a) T.
    (b) T.
    (c) T.
    (d) F.
    (e) T.

47. (a) F. Autistic children fail to show the usual relatedness
           to their parents and other people.
    (b) T.

(c) F. Dyslexia is usually apparent by age 7.
(d) F. Disintegrative psychosis usually begins between ages 3 and 5.
(e) T.

48. (a) T.
(b) F.
(c) T.
(d) T.
(e) F.
Item (e) suggests cognitive impairment more likely to be due to a dementing process than depression.

49. (a) F.
(b) F.
(c) F.
(d) T.
(e) T.

50. (a) T.
(b) T.
(c) T.
(d) T.
(e) F. Behaviour modification helps in some patients.

Reference

Kinsey, A. C., Pomeroy, W. B. and Martin, C. E. (1948) 'Sexual behaviour in the human male' Philadelphia, W. B. Saunders.

PMPs/ORAL EXAMINATION

PMPs – the Oral Examination

This part of the practical examination is a test of communication and judgement.

The clinical case histories will be drawn from any area of psychiatry. Most of them are related to your clinical experience. You may have encountered some of them during your training.

You will be asked about 3 or 4 case histories on different clinical topics.

Listen carefully to the examiners. If you are not clear about the question, do ask them gently to repeat it, but do not keep asking to repeat each question.

Use all the given information in trying to understand the case histories.

Try to be as eclectic as possible. Say if there is inadequate information to work on, and suggest how you will go about obtaining the necessary information.

Do not try to cross-question the examiners even if you do not agree with the question asked or if it appears silly to you.

Try to give a balanced answer, but don't be afraid if you are sure of a particular type of treatment; be prepared to argue about it constructively.

If you get bogged down in one of the questions, say honestly that you do not know the answer. The examiners will then probably move on to the next question.

Think about the chronology or sequence of likely events. Think both longitudinally as well as laterally.

Remember the importance of multi-disciplinary teamwork.

In brief, your answers should be based on the *following outline*:

- General opening/special features.
- Sources of history.
- History taking and mental state examination.

- Explanation of symptoms, i.e. diagnosis and differential diagnosis.
- Management plan.
- Prognosis: short-term and long-term.

The answers given are an attempt to provide a model or framework to use in dealing with the questions. There is room for differences of opinion, as there are variations in clinical practice around the country. Some of the answers may appear over-inclusive. This is a deliberate attempt to give the examinees as much information as possible.

PATIENT MANAGEMENT PROBLEMS

1. A 25-year-old female was brought to your local accident and emergency department following an overdose and self-inflicted injuries to her wrists and forearms. She refuses to cooperate with the Casualty Officer. You are invited to assist in the situation. How would you deal with it?

Assessment

- History from the Casualty Officer of the overdose and self-inflicted injuries.
- From a reliable informant about the current situation, past behaviour and relevant psychiatric illness.

Interview with the patient

- Introduce myself to the patient and explain the purpose of my involvement.
- Acknowledge to the patient that I am aware of the problems and her non-cooperation.
- Detailed assessment of her suicidal potentials:
  - reasons for the present deliberate self-harm;
  - psychiatric illness – present/past;
  - alcohol/drug abuse;
  - physical illness;
  - premorbid personality;
  - social circumstances;
  - recent life events;
  - reasons for non-cooperation; e.g. still wanting to die.

Management

Depends on the assessment of the problem and patient's cooperation.

- Obviously, she has been uncooperative so far.
- Even after persuasion, if she is still uncooperative, admission to the psychiatric unit might be arranged under provisions of the Mental Health Act for serious suicidal intent.
- Such an admission will take place either under Emergency Order (Section 4 or equivalent) or Assessment Order (Section 2 or equivalent).
- If the suicide risk is not considered to be of a serious nature, and the patient still refuses to cooperate, she may be allowed to leave the hospital.
- I would notify her general practitioner and next of kin as soon as possible.
- Follow-up in the Out-patient Clinic or Day Hospital would be arranged.
- No legal provision is available to impose treatment for physical problems.

2. A middle-aged Asian woman, currently an in-patient for the treatment of paranoid schizophrenia, has experienced difficulties with eating and staying still. You are on call and are requested to assess her condition. She also requests leave for the weekend. You notice rhythmic movements of her lips and tongue. What steps would you take to assist this patient?

Assessment

- History from the nursing staff, patient and other informants.
- Type of onset.
- Duration of the symptoms in relation to the drug therapy.
- Information from the case notes regarding the past history of similar problems and the response to treatment.

- Current drug therapy; e.g. type of drug, its dosage, route of administration, duration, etc.
- Mental state examination.
- Physical examination, including gait, reflexes, muscle tone, eye muscles.

Management

- It seems that the patient has developed tardive dyskinesia and akathisia as a result of drug therapy for schizophrenia.
- Depending on her mental state, the pharmacological treatment would be as follows:
  - reduce the dosage of her neuroleptic drugs, or no change at all;
  - addition (if not already prescribed) of anti-Parkinsonian drug, preferably by an intra-muscular route, followed by regular oral administration until her symptoms are resolved.
- Permission for weekend leave will depend on her mental state, the severity of her side-effects and family support. In view of the present problem, it would be advisable for her to stay on the ward for further observation.

3. A 35-year-old, married, Caucasian mother of 5 children under the age of 10 years presents with a long history of bipolar affective disorder and a dislike of sex. She washes all the bed linen and takes a bath after sexual intercourse with her husband. She refuses to take contraceptive measures or have sterilization on religious grounds. She is now 3 months pregnant and has stopped her lithium carbonate just after missing her period. Discuss briefly the main points of your assessment and subsequent management.

Assessment

- Detailed history of her problems, mainly ruminations, rituals, dislike of sex, mood changes.

- Was the pregnancy planned or unplanned, and what would she like to do about it?
- See her husband and obtain further information, especially about their marital relationship, children, past psychiatric history.
- Information from her case notes, general practitioner and other reliable sources regarding any post-natal psychiatric disorders and their response to treatment, especially lithium therapy.
- Likelihood of future pregnancies.

Management

- Will largely depend on her present mental state, and her wishes about her pregnancy.
- Observation in Out-patient Clinic, visits by community psychiatric nurse and health visitor.
- If she wishes to continue with the pregnancy, it is most advisable not to recommence on lithium carbonate.
- Advice about prevention of future pregnancies, including vasectomy for her husband.
- Explanation about the nature of bipolar affective disorder.
- Behaviour modification for her ritualistic behaviour.
- Marital therapy will be necessary.
- Support for children.

4. A 45-year-old single man of no fixed abode attends your Out-patient Clinic. He has a long history of psychotic illness and a prison record for various offences, including burglary, theft, assault, etc. Most recently, he pleaded to charges of theft of a prescription pad from his general practitioner's surgery, but he was let off lightly by the court. He refuses to take his medication, including a depot injection. How would you assess his condition? What do you think is the best course of action to manage the current situation?

Assessment

- History from the patient himself, general practitioner, family (if any), probation officer and previous case notes regarding the past psychiatric illness and its response to treatment and the criminal record.
- Social support.
- Drug abuse of illicit drugs and prescribed drugs like benzodiazepines.
- Level of insight.
- Motivation to change for the better.
- Dangerousness and risk of further criminal behaviour.
- Mental state examination.
- Risk to his health and safety and/or to the safety of the public.

Management

This will depend upon the underlying psychiatric disorder and the deviant personality. There are various diagnostic possibilities; e.g. paranoid schizophrenia, paranoid disorder, drug-induced paranoid psychosis, inadequate and/or psychopathic personality disorder.

If the patient is uncooperative with the assessment, it will be difficult to prepare a treatment plan. The courts have already dealt with him leniently, which does not help the present situation.

The best course of action, in my opinion, is to arrange for a Treatment Order under the current provisions of the Mental Health Act for the following reasons:

- Long history of psychiatric illness.
- Refusal to cooperate with voluntary treatment.
- He is certainly a risk to his own health and safety.
- He is of no fixed abode.
- His criminal behaviour might be associated with his psychiatric illness.
- There is an absence of any legal provisions to treat him compulsorily in the community.

5. You are presented with a 40-year-old woman with 6
   children under the age of 15 years. Her husband who is 15
   years her senior, is unemployed and abuses alcohol. She
   looks undernourished and feels scared for no apparent
   reason. She also complains of disturbed sleep for the past 3
   months. Discuss the diagnostic possibilities and prognosis
   in this case.

Differential diagnosis

The following should be considered.
(a) *Organic/physical illness*
   e.g. thyrotoxicosis, diabetes mellitus,
        pulmonary tuberculosis,
        anaemia – iron deficiency;
              B12 deficiency;
              folic deficiency.
(b) *Psychiatric illness*
   - Depression.
   - Anxiety state (generalized anxiety disorder).
   - Panic disorder.
   - Anorexia nervosa.
   - Alcohol abuse.
   - Benzodiazepine dependence.

Prognosis

(a) *Short-term prognosis*
   This will depend on:
   - The underlying diagnosis, associated factors like
     stress generated by the alcoholic husband, financial
     difficulties, marital disharmony.
   - Response to treatment, which may necessitate
     hospitalization.
   - Patient's motivation and cooperation with treatment.
(b) *Long-term prognosis*
   In addition to the factors mentioned above, it will also
   depend on:

- Husband's willingness and ability to stop drinking.
- Marital therapy.
- Improvement in the financial circumstances.

6. A 45-year-old man living in a staffed hostel has become
   uncooperative, irritable and verbally aggressive towards
   other people over the past 2 weeks. His sleep has been
   disturbed, and in fact he has spent less time asleep. You are
   contacted by the community psychiatric nurse for advice
   and further management of this case. What steps would
   you take in dealing with this situation?

   To deal with the above situation, it is necessary to make
   an assessment and prepare a treatment plan.

Assessment

- More information about his present condition and
  behaviour from the community psychiatric nurse, and
  the hostel staff.
- Relatives (if any).
- Mitigating circumstances; e.g. stress, relationship with
  staff and residents at the hostel.
- Compliance with his prescribed medication.
- Effect of his behaviour on himself and others.
- Relapse or recurrence of his illness.
- Alcohol or drug abuse.
- Serum level of lithium carbonate, if applicable.

Treatment plan

Obviously it will depend on the underlying psychiatric
illness. It is most likely that he is suffering from an affective
or psychotic illness like bipolar illness, schizo-affective
disorder or schizophrenia.
(a) *Immediate advice*
   - To administer oral and/or intra-muscular dosage of a
     neuroleptic drug like haloperidol.

- Alternatively, to administer a dosage of clopenthixol
  acuphase which, given intra-muscularly, might be
  most appropriate if the patient is cooperative.
- To notify the patient's general practitioner.

(b) *Subsequent management*
  - To arrange to see him as soon as possible.
  - To study the hospital notes and establish an
    understanding of his problem.
  - To review his medication if necessary.
  - To liaise with the hostel staff and community
    psychiatric nurse and provide support to them.
  - To consider hospitalization to stabilize his condition
    if the hostel staff cannot manage him.

7. You are approached informally by the Clinical Director of
the Surgical Services in your hospital. He is concerned
about a consultant surgeon colleague who has become
depressed following recent death of his wife. The surgeon
drinks alcohol to an excess even at work and is unwilling to
see a psychiatrist. How would you assist the Clinical
Director? What do you think is most likely to happen in
this case?

Two main issues

(a) To assist an unwilling colleague.
(b) Prognosis: both short-term and long-term.

(a) As the surgeon is unwilling to see a psychiatrist, the
assessment of his problems will depend largely on
information obtained from other sources, for example:
  - Clinical Director.
  - Family members.
  - General practitioner, if possible.
  There are ethical issues like speaking with the patient's
  relatives, general practitioner, Clinical Director and
  other people without his knowledge and permission.
  - Information about the surgeon's wife's last illness
    and circumstances of her death.

- Information about onset, duration and severity of depression and drinking, suicidal attempts/thoughts, if any.
- Behaviour with colleagues.
- Unauthorized absence from work, cancellations of Out-patient Clinics and operating lists.
- Try to see the surgeon and reassure him about confidentiality.
- Encourage the Clinical Director to liaise with the surgeon's general practitioner if he is still unwilling to cooperate with an informal approach.
- Approach the National Counselling Service for Sick Doctors (an independent confidential service) – telephone 071-935-5982.

Prognosis

It is very difficult to predict the outcome, as the patient is unwilling to cooperate with the assessment and management of his problems. However, I would like to think that he would receive the most appropriate treatment, achieve maximum improvement and relieve others of their concerns about him.

- In the view of the current status of Clinical Director and Medical Director, does the Three Wise Men still operate?
- Could the surgeon sue for libel if enquiries were made about him implying that he might have a drink problem?

8. You are asked by a local general practitioner to see a 35-year-old female who is feeling suicidally depressed. She is 8 weeks pregnant and has 5 children between the ages of 2 and 15. Her husband is unemployed and is threatening to leave her. She is ambivalent about her pregnancy. What advice would you give to the general practitioner? How would you arrive at your advice?

Advice to general practitioner

(a) Suicidal risk.
(b) Management of depression.
(c) Continuation/termination of pregnancy.
(d) Contraception/sterilization to prevent an unwanted future pregnancy.
(e) Marital therapy.

Process of assessment to provide the advice

Interview both partners separately and together.
- History, especially past psychiatric history.
- Mental state examination.
- Was the pregnancy planned or unplanned?
- What contraceptive measures were taken?
- Why is she ambivalent about the pregnancy?
- What does he think about the pregnancy?
- Explore the marital disharmony.
- Implications of continuing/discontinuing the pregnancy.
- Implications of pharmacological treatment (if necessary).
- Effect of her depression and marital disharmony on children.
- Do they want any more children (already have 5 and probably 6 in the near future)?
- If she is still ambivalent about pregnancy, she may be referred for specialist counselling as available in most obstetric departments.

9. A 46-year-old single male stays in a hostel on 'trial' to assess his suitability for admission to the hostel. He has refused to take his fortnightly depot injection for the past 2 months. His mental state has deteriorated significantly over the past 2 weeks. The hostel staff and his general practitioner are concerned about him and request your help. How would you manage this situation?

Assessment

- History of his present condition from the patient (if he is cooperative), the hostel staff, general practitioner, community psychiatric nurse, family (if any), fellow residents of the hostel.
- Case notes regarding past psychiatric history; e.g. diagnosis, hospital admissions, response to treatment.
- Visit the patient and explore why he refuses to take his medication; e.g. side-effects, loss of insight, peer pressure.
- Identify stressors.
- Previous history of non-cooperation and methods used to manage it.
- Present mental state examination.

Management

This will depend on various factors.
- It is clear that the patient's mental state has deteriorated mainly due to a relapse in his schizophrenic illness.
- Persuade him to recommence on his depot injections and oral neuroleptic drugs (to bring about a quick recovery).
- Explain the consequences of his non-cooperation with prescribed treatment; e.g. loss of placement at the hostel.
- If he still refuses to cooperate at the hostel, a further period of observation will be necessary until an informal or a compulsory admission to the local Psychiatric Unit is warranted.

10. You are asked to see a 70-year-old woman who has been taking diazepam for the past 20 years. She is alert but has mild lapses in her short-term memory. She would like to stop taking her drug, but is unable to do so. Her 75-year-old husband is showing some evidence of Alzheimer's disease. Explain how you would deal with this patient.

Assessment

History
- Benzodiazepine dependence (diazepam dosage, tolerance, withdrawal symptoms in the past).
- Circumstances which initiated and maintained her dependence on diazepam.
- Current stressors; e.g. burden of looking after her husband.
- Husband's condition; i.e. Alzheimer's disease.
- Past psychiatric history.
- Concomitant physical illness and drugs.

Mental state examination

- She is showing signs of impairment of short-term memory which may be due to diazepam.
- Look for signs/symptoms of a dementing disorder and other disorders like generalized anxiety disorder and depression.

Management

- Ethical questions – such as whether or not she should stop taking diazepam – should be considered.
- Obviously, she is motivated to stop taking it, but is under stress.
- Consider implications of stopping diazepam, e.g., prolonged withdrawal syndrome, return of the original condition and increased difficulties in managing her life.
- If it is decided to stop diazepam, it will need to be done in steps. Replacement with a selective serotonin re-uptake inhibitor drug will be appropriate.
- If it is decided not to stop, the *status quo* should be maintained.
- Practical help.
- Respite/phased care for her husband in a Psychogeriatric Unit.

- Day care for both.
- Liaison with her general practitioner and other agencies.

11. You are on call for your hospital. The ward manager bleeps you with an urgent problem, telling you that an informally admitted, depressed patient wants to leave the ward against his advice. How would you assess and deal with this patient?

Assessment

- History from the ward staff, patient, family and case notes. Note his age, sex, marital status, severity of depression, concomitant physical illness, suicidal intention, past suicidal attempts, alcohol or drug abuse.
- Family support.
- Reasons for leaving the ward.
- Previous hospitalization for depression and response to treatment, including electroconvulsive therapy.

Management

- After an assessment of the patient's condition, there are various options:
  (a) discussion with the senior doctor on call or the patient's own responsible medical officer;
  (b) persuading the patient to continue with the in-patient treatment;
  (c) if it is not possible to do so, there may be grounds to detain the patient under the Mental Health Act (e.g. suicidal behaviour).
- Therapeutic measures, along with close observation.

12. A 50-year-old male civil servant whose driver's licence was suspended following a road traffic accident is suffering from a bipolar affective disorder. The local driver's licence office requests a medical report to assess his fitness to drive. Explain how you would deal with this request.

Assessment

- History from the patient, family, general practitioner, and case notes of present and previous psychiatric illness, especially bipolar affective disorder.
- Circumstances of the road traffic accident and injuries/damage sustained by all parties concerned.
- Mental state examination.
- History of physical disorders like diabetes mellitus, heart diseases or epilepsy which may impair his fitness to drive.
- Effects of his psychotropic drugs, including adverse effects.
- Reasons for suspension of his licence.

Medical report

This should include the following information:
- Current mental state.
- Response to treatment.
- Adverse effects of drug treatment, if any.
- Prognosis.
- Fitness/unfitness to drive, based on the above information and implications on his livelihood, and personal and public safety.

13. A 70-year-old widow was recently admitted for psychiatric assessment. It was then felt that she would not be able to manage on her own at her home and would need sheltered accommodation. However, there is a disagreement in the multi-disciplinary team regarding her disposal. Discuss how, as a doctor in charge of the patient, you would deal with this situation.

   - Explore the reasons for disagreement with the professionals concerned; e.g. is the disagreement about the patient's ability to look after herself or about the suitability of accommodation?
   - Review the case thoroughly to identify if anything was missed at the original meeting.

- Discuss this matter with her family (if any), and seek their views.
- Under the provisions of the NHS and Community Care Act 1990, it is essential to arrange a joint assessment by Health and Social Services and to agree to the funding of her placement.
- Try to resolve the disagreement amicably, if possible.
- Look at alternatives to the original proposal; e.g.
  (a) home care with support;
  (b) care with family, if appropriate;
  (c) hospital care.
- Don't forget to consider the patient's wishes, which are of paramount importance.
- Having gone through all available informal options to resolve the disagreement, if there is still no resolution, a formal approach will be required.

14. You are seeing a young male in the Accident and Emergency Department. Following your assessment, you believe that this patient requires compulsory admission to the Psychiatric Unit. The approved social worker is of the contrary opinion. Discuss how you would manage this situation.

   An assessment has been made to consider compulsory admission because:
   (a) the patient is considered mentally disordered or is suspected to be so;
   (b) he is a danger to his health or safety or to the safety of other people;
   (c) He is unwilling to cooperate with informal admission.
- Seek further explanations from the approved social worker regarding his or her disagreement with your assessment.
- Seek an opinion from another doctor, preferably the patient's general practitioner, and/or the senior doctor (who is approved under a section of the Mental Health Act).
- Seek an opinion from the nearest relative or the next of kin regarding the patient's condition.

- If there is still disagreement with the approved social worker, 2 options are available:
  - (i) do nothing more and abdicate the responsibility of care to Social Services;
  - (ii) invite the nearest relative to apply to the hospital managers on the basis of 1 or 2 medical recommendations. (This is not regarded as good clinical practice.)

15. You are asked to see a patient following his admission to a medical ward who is almost completely mute. The physician would like you to assess him and then transfer him to the psychiatric ward. How would you proceed and manage this request?

   The physician confirms that the patient is physically fit to be transferred to the psychiatric ward. I therefore assume that organic causes of mutism have been ruled out.

Assessment

- History from the staff, family, general practitioner or other informants (if available) regarding age, sex, marital status, past psychiatric illness, premorbid personality.
- Visit the patient on the medical ward.
- Observe whether the patient is alert and follows what is happening around him.
- Note whether or not the patient is able to communicate in writing.
- Observe whether the mutism is associated with loss of bodily movements.
- Mental state examination is difficult due to absence of speech.
- Try to rule out functional causes of mutism; e.g. schizophrenia, depression, hysteria.
- Try to obtain information from the Munchausen Register (if it exists at the hospital and also neighbouring hospitals).

Management

- Transfer the patient to the psychiatric ward for further assessment.

16. A 45-year-old married woman was referred to you by her general practitioner for a psychiatric assessment. She complains that she was sexually abused by her father's best friend at the age of 11. She requests help. How would you assist this patient?

Assessment

- History from the patient, husband, general practitioner and other relevant sources such as her parents.
- Details about her alleged abuse, including whether sexual intercourse took place or not.
- Whether her parents, especially her father, knew about her ordeal.
- Whether or not the alleged abuser is alive.
- When did she first realize that she was sexually abused?
- What are the effects of abuse on her mental health and marital life?
- How does her husband view her problem, and what support does he offer her?
- Are there any sexual difficulties in her marriage?
- Her feelings about being abused.
- Evidence of any major psychiatric disorders such as depression.
- Hatred of men.
- Risk of abuse of her children.
- Mental state examination will be vital in assessing her condition.

Management

- Treatment of concomitant psychiatric disorder, if any.
- Individual psychotherapy.

- Group psychotherapy might be more appropriate, if available.
- Marital therapy should be considered, if necessary.

17. You suspect that there is an incestuous relationship between a man and his 14-year-old stepdaughter. The girl's mother has noticed some kind of disturbance in her behaviour and is worried about her frequent unauthorized absence from school. Discuss briefly what steps you would take to assess the situation and help the family.

Assessment

History from the girl, mother, stepfather, headteacher or tutor about:
- Marital breakdown.
- Social isolation.
- Over-crowded conditions; sharing bedrooms.
- Excessive drinking and antisocial personality of the stepfather.
- Behaviour at school, especially truancy.
- Unexplained suicidal attempts.
- Any other children at risk or being abused.
- Physical examination of the girl, including collection of specimens from the genital and other regions if intercourse has taken place within 72 hours.

Mental state examination

- Depressed mood.
- Low self-esteem.

Management

(a) Measures to protect the child:
  - Notify Social Services, police.
  - Case conference to be arranged by the social worker.

- The girl's name may be put on the At Risk Register.
- The separation of the girl from her family if incest is established is most appropriate.
- The stepfather may face criminal charges.

(b) The family might need help with their emotional problems through the Child and Family Psychiatric Services.

(c) Counselling for the girl.

(d) Liaison with the school educational psychologist.

18. A 65-year-old man was picked up by highway police and brought to the local general hospital. He was admitted for close observation. The physician in charge of his care requests a psychiatric assessment. Outline the steps you would take to make a thorough assessment.

Assessment

History from police, patient, relatives, general practitioner, neighbours, staff of a care home (if applicable).
- Wandering behaviour.
- Psychiatric disorder.
- Physical disorder, head injury.
- Drugs.
- Premorbid personality.
- Life events.

Mental state examination

- Level of consciousness.
- General behaviour.
- Disorders of perceptions/thoughts.
- Cognitive functions.
- Judgement insight.
- General knowledge.

It may be necessary to test linguistic, visuospatial and other high cortical functions.

- Physical examination, including neurological assessment along with that of vision and hearing.
- Investigations to rule out various conditions like diabetes mellitus, heart disease, infections, etc.

Diagnosis/differential diagnosis should be arrived at following the above procedures.

19. You are asked to see a middle-aged housewife at her home. She has been house-bound for a long time. Her husband and children find it difficult to enjoy their family and social life. Explain how you would assess and manage this woman.

Assessment

History from the patient, husband, children and the general practitioner.
- Anxiety symptoms.
- Panic attacks.
- Anxious cognitions about fainting and loss of control.
- Situations which provoke anxiety and avoidance.
- Anticipatory anxiety.
- Depressive symptoms, depersonalization and obsessional thoughts.
- Onset and course of the above symptoms.
- Predisposing, precipitating and maintaining factors.
- How and why the family and social life is affected.

Diagnosis

Agoraphobia.

Differential diagnosis

- Generalized anxiety disorder.
- Social phobic disorder.
- Depressive disorder.
- Paranoid disorder.

Management

- Treatment of choice – behaviour therapy combined with exposure to phobic situations with training in coping with panic attacks.
- Drug therapy – secondary to behaviour therapy, anxiolytic and antidepressant drugs to treat concomitant symptoms.

20. You are working on an acute admission ward. You are confronted with a severely depressed patient who was admitted following a suicide attempt. He refuses to eat, drink or cooperate with the treatment. Discuss how you would manage this patient.

Assessment of the risk of suicide

- History from the case notes, patient, family.
- Previous history of depression or other psychiatric disorder.
- Response to treatment, including electroconvulsive therapy.
- Other risk factors; e.g. age, sex, marital status, alcohol or drug abuse, physical illness, bereavement.
- Physical status, including blood screening, ECG and chest X-ray.

Management

(a) *Informal approach*:
  - Persuade the patient; use family support if available.
  - Physical treatment like intra-venous hyper-alimentation.
  - Antidepressant drugs.
  - Emergency electroconvulsive therapy under the common law of Parliament.

(b) *Formal approach*:
  - If the patient still refuses to cooperate and there is considered to be a serious risk to his health and/or safety, he should be placed under a Treatment Order of the Mental Health Act.
  - Second opinion from Mental Health Act Commission or equivalent body.
  - The above physical methods of treatment should be offered.

21. You are asked by a local general practitioner to see a housewife whose family is 'fed up' with her, because she does not allow visitors to the home. She spends a lot of time cleaning and tidying up the house. Discuss what steps you would take to assess and manage her condition.

Assessment

History from patient, husband, children, friends, general practitioner regarding origin, duration and progress of the following:
- How does she see her problems?
- What happens if people come to her house?
- Fear of dirt, contamination, etc.
- Obsessional thoughts, doubts.
- Ruminations, rituals.
- Obsessional slowness and phobia.
- Mental state examination.

Diagnosis

- Obsessive compulsive disorder.

Differential diagnosis

- Generalized anxiety disorder.
- Panic disorder.

- Phobic disorder.
- Depression.
- Schizophrenia.
- Organic cerebral disorder (e.g. encephalitis lethargica).

Management

- Explanation of the symptoms.
- Encourage the family to adopt a firm but sympathetic attitude to the patient.
- Drugs: anxiolytic and/or antidepressant drugs may be of some value.
- Response prevention and exposure to environmental cues that increase them.
- Thought stopping.
- Supportive psychotherapy.

22. A 75-year-old female patient suffering from paranoid schizophrenia is considered ready for discharge to a residential care home. She has developed a huge prolapse of the rectum over the last few years, but she does not acknowledge the problem and refuses to give her consent for a surgical operation. Her next of kin are willing to give written consent on her behalf. Discuss how you would manage her proposed discharge from the hospital.

Main issues

(a) Proposed discharge to a home for residential care.
(b) Dealing with the surgical condition.

Assessment

- History from the patient, next of kin and the ward staff

about the prolapse of the rectum; e.g. duration, size, complications, etc.
- Re-assessment of her mental state.
- Explore why the patient does not acknowledge the problem when it is evident to everyone else.
- It is apparent that she does not realize the seriousness of her surgical condition even though she knows that she has a problem.
- She is considered ready for discharge to a residential care home where the staff are probably aware of her problems.
- Enquire if she has been seen by the surgical specialist, and if so, seek his opinion.
- Explore if she is to continue voluntarily with the psychiatric treatment after her discharge from hospital.

Management

- It may be that her discharge from hospital is dependent on the surgical repair of the rectal prolapse.
- Discuss the surgical problem with the staff at the residential care home, and the patient's blatant refusal to receive appropriate treatment.
- Share your concern with the patient's next of kin, who are prepared to give consent on her behalf. From a legal point of view, only the patient's consent is required for the surgical operation necessary in this case.
- No legal provisions exist to assist the present situation, as it is not considered a life-threatening condition.
- Explain to the patient the potential dangers of her refusal to receive surgical treatment, and document.
- Write about your concern in case notes.
- If the residential care home is willing to accept her in her present condition, the proposed discharge should go ahead.
- Notify the general practitioner about problems faced with this patient and advise him or her to review them in the future.
- If, however, the home is unable to accept her, she should stay in hospital until a suitable alternative is available.

23. You are seeing a middle-aged patient in your Out-patient Clinic at the request of his general practitioner, who is concerned about his long absence from work. The patient admits to drinking alcohol to excess and spanking his wife's bottom in order to achieve sexual arousal. He is trying, without success, to have a baby. Discuss the differential diagnosis and management of this case.

Differential diagnosis

- Alcohol abuse.
- Depression (major depressive disorder).
- Bipolar affective disorder.
- Generalized anxiety disorder.
- Obsessive compulsive disorder.
- Sexual sadism.

Management

It depends on assessment of the underlying condition, which will require history taking and appropriate investigations.

History should be obtained from the patient, wife and employers.
- All the above differential diagnoses should be considered as a strong possibility.

Enquiry regarding:

- Type of work.
- Position of responsibility.
- Length of absence of work.
- Any informal/formal warning received.
- Relationships with wife, who might be masochist and cooperate with the patient.
- Sexual history/fantasies.
- Motivation to change.

212 The Complete MRCPsych Part II

- Past psychiatric/medical history.
- Investigations for infertility.

Treatment plan

- Detoxification for alcohol abuse.
- Treatment of concomitant psychiatric disorder.
- Marital therapy if indicated.
- Sex therapy.
- Aim at return to work.

24. The police picked up a 28-year-old, dishevelled and unkempt man on a cold winter night. He claimed that he is a psychiatric registrar at your hospital. The police believed that he was deluded, and a danger to himself and to the public. You are asked to visit him at the police station, confirm his identity and deal with the situation.

Assessment

- First of all, inform the senior medical staff on call and discuss the case before visiting him at the police station.
- Enquire from the police whether he is detained under an order of the Mental Health Act 1983.
- Invite the approved social worker to join you to assess the patient.
- Identify him correctly.
- History from the patient, family (if available), general practitioner and other reliable informants.
- Mental state examination.
- Assessment of danger to himself and/or others.

Management

- Very difficult situation if he is a colleague.
- Admission for observation and further assessment, either on an informal or formal basis if indicated.

- Admission should be considered to another hospital outside the rotational training scheme.
- If admission is not warranted, an out-patient follow-up should be arranged in another area.
- Liaise with his general practitioner and family as soon as possible.

25. A 40-year-old, married, female schoolteacher was involved in a road traffic accident while going to work. She has lost all her confidence and is unable to attend to her work following the accident. Her solicitors have advised her to claim compensation from the third party. You are requested to see her and prepare a psychiatric report. Explain how you would assist this woman and her solicitors.

Assessment

History from the patient, general practitioner, solicitors, family and school about the patient's clinical problems, including onset, duration and severity.
- Information about the road traffic accident and the patient's disability.
- Past psychiatric/medical history.
- Premorbid personality.
- What compensation is being sought and how would it help her and her family.

Diagnosis

Post traumatic stress disorder.

Differential diagnosis

(a) *Organic conditions*:
   - Head injury.
   - Alcohol dependence.
   - Drug dependence.

(b) *Psychiatric disorders*:
- Factitious disorder.
- Malingering.
- Adjustment reaction.
- Borderline personality disorder.
- Schizophrenia.
- Depression.
- Panic disorder.
- Generalized anxiety disorder.

Diagnosis of post-traumatic stress disorder depends on such diagnostic features as:
- The traumatic event is persistently experienced in a variety of ways.
- Persistent avoidance of stimuli associated with the trauma.
- Persistent symptoms of increased arousal.

Psychiatric report will include

- Assessment of the psychiatric symptoms and the patient's disability.
- Causal relationship of her symptoms to the road traffic accident.
- Prognosis, short-term and long-term.
- Possibility of successful return to work.
- Treatment required:
  - pharmacological;
  - psychotherapy: individual therapy;
                    group therapy;
                    family therapy.

26. You have been informed by your ward manager that one of your patients was found dead in his room. How would you deal with this situation?

Main issues

(a) Certifying the death, notifying the police and coroner.

(b) Breaking the news to the family and supporting them.
(c) Investigation into the death.
(d) Support to the staff and patients.

(a) *Certifying the death*:
  - If the cause of death was obvious, provide the death certificate.
  - If the death occurred in suspicious circumstances or was unnatural, the coroner must be notified.
  - The coroner will arrange for the post mortem and an inquest, if considered necessary.
  - Notify the police if unlawful activity is suspected.

(b) *Breaking the news to the family*:
This is the most delicate issue, which requires consideration and the utmost care.
  - If the relatives are on the telephone, contact them immediately.
  - If they are not on the phone or are not available, the police should be invited to offer assistance in breaking the news.
  - Provide support to the family before, during and after the funeral.

(c) *Investigation into the death*:
  - Inform the senior medical staff.
  - Obtain information from the staff and witnesses (if any) about the mode of death, and prepare a detailed report.
  - Consider the possibility of suicide.
  - Be prepared to assist an official investigation carried out by the hospital managers, coroner and police, and libel and/or action by the family.

(d) *Support to staff and patients*:
  - Arrange meetings with staff and patients to allow them to ventilate their feelings.
  - Invite the hospital chaplain, who might be able to assist in the situation.

27. You are confronted with a 45-year-old married West Indian man who is detained under section 37/41 of the Mental Health Act 1983. He has appealed to the Mental Health Review Tribunal for his discharge. You are asked by your consultant to prepare a report for the Tribunal. How would you proceed in this case?

- Introduce yourself, and explain why you are preparing the report.
- Obtain as much information as possible from various sources, including his family.
- Read the details about index offence(s) and also refer to the psychiatric reports prepared at the time of the court appearance.
- Progress during the present admission – discuss with the relevant staff and family.
- Establish whether there is a time limit imposed on his Restriction Order.
- Current psychiatric diagnosis, length of stay.
- Response to various treatments, including pharmacological methods.
- Escorted/unescorted leave granted or not? Has he been allowed to go outside hospital, visit his family?
- Current status of relationship with his family, especially wife and children.
- Patient's own view about release from Restriction Order.
- Whether there is any guilt or remorse about his past action.
- Whether he is willing to stay in hospital as an informal patient.
- Whether he expects an immediate absolute discharge from the hospital, or whether he should remain under the order until there is a review.
- Recommendations depend on the above information.
- Liaise with the social worker, probation officer, community psychiatric nurse, etc.
- Decide whether he is ready for discharge or not. If not, give reasons; e.g. mentally unwell, lack of insight, being a danger to himself and/or others.

- If he is considered ready for discharge, qualify your view by giving additional information; e.g. living at staffed hostel, group home, independent council accommodation, etc.
- Need for medication, day care.
- Family's wishes to take him home or not.
- Follow-up by social worker, community psychiatric nurse or other agency as seen appropriate.
- Give information about his prognosis.

28. You are asked by a local general practitioner to see a 32-year-old, married, Asian woman who has been behaving in a childish way. She carries her food and a flask of water with her all the time. Her family has noticed that she washes her hands several times a day. She refuses to see you. What might be your plan to deal with this patient?

It is usually difficult to interview a patient if she refuses to cooperate. In this particular case, it is very important to obtain all the available information from other sources. If the patient refuses to give permission to consult her husband and other members of the family, the problem becomes even more difficult. However, it might be necessary to talk to her husband and/or family members, especially her mother-in-law, in complete confidence in order to obtain the necessary information.

Information is required about

- What constitutes childish behaviour and its duration?
- Patient's understanding regarding carrying food and water all the time and repeated hand washing.
- Any other behaviour which is considered excessive and abnormal.
- Effects of patient's behaviour and her relationship within the family and with children (if any).
- Family structure and dynamics.
- Patient's level of insight, which already appears to be limited.

- Stressful life events.
- Her marriage, psychosexual history, weight and body image.
- Past psychiatric history of the patient and her family members.

Diagnostic possibilities

- Schizophrenia.
- Depression.
- Obsessive compulsive disorder.
- Anorexia nervosa.
- Bulimia nervosa.
- Malingering.
- Inadequate personality disorder.

Further actions

- Try to persuade the patient to discuss her problems by involving her parents if they are willing and available.
- Ask her if she prefers to talk to a woman who speaks an Asian language.
- If all the above efforts fail, I would consider an assessment in hospital under Section 2 of the Mental Health Act 1983 if there are grounds for such an action.

29. You are asked to accompany your consultant to visit a 69-year-old, conditionally discharged transsexual man in a special hospital. One of the conditions of his discharge requires him to go to a community-based facility in your catchment area. Explain how you would assess him and what the after-care plan should consist of.

   - First of all, discuss your thoughts with your consultant and obtain the guidance you might feel you need.
   - Carefully read the judgement delivered by the Mental Health Review Tribunal and try to understand its implications for your resources and service.

- Enquire if any member of staff at your hospital was involved in dealing with the Tribunal.
- Discuss the case with patient's responsible medical officer and other staff at the special hospital.
- Detailed history of index offence(s), if applicable, length of current admission and previous admissions to special and other psychiatric hospitals.
- Present mental state.
- Present treatment programme.
- Present level of social functioning; e.g. self-care, daily living skills, etc.
- Physical health.
- Treatment received for transsexuality.
- Whether the patient is allowed to cross-dress all the time, a little of the time or not at all.

The patient's wishes are of paramount importance in this particular case:

- Does he want to live the rest of his life as a woman?
- Where would he like to live?
- Contact with family, if applicable.

The Tribunal has considered him fit for conditional discharge and not a danger to himself and/or the public. The accommodation required will depend on the Tribunal's directions.

- Consider any previous attempts to resettle this man in the community.
- Consider the special toilet and bath facilities he will need if he chooses to live as a woman.

Follow-up arrangement

- Out-patient Clinic.
- Domiciliary support.
- Day care.
- Attendance at gender clinic.
- Contact with an organization for transsexuals.
- Social worker follow-up if community psychiatric nurse is required.

Back-up support from

- Special hospital.
- Regional Secure Unit.
- Local Secure Unit.

30. You are asked to see a 15-year-old girl in your Accident and Emergency Department. She has been reported to be worried about catching HIV and AIDS. She was bullied in her school for about 6 months until recently. Her parents are concerned about her. How would you assess this young girl? What are the possible differential diagnoses?

History

Obtain her history from the patient and her parents.
- Try to ascertain why she has attended the hospital and whether she has discussed this matter with her general practitioner.
- Source of referral; e.g. self or a third party.
- Is there a history of deliberate self-harm?
- Life events.
- Details of her bullying experience.
- Explore her concerns about her fears; i.e. catching HIV and AIDS.
- Enquire about her psychosexual history, peer group pressure, sibling rivalry, school work.
- A detailed mental state examination should reveal further information.

Differential diagnosis should include

- Depression.
- Stress reaction.
- Obsessive compulsive disorder.
- Generalized anxiety disorder.
- Panic disorder.

GUIDELINES FOR THE CLINICAL EXAMINATION

The examination

The clinical examination is the most important part of the whole MRCPsych Part II examination, as it is necessary to pass in order to achieve success in the examination. It is not dissimilar to a good clinical ward round. The examinee is allowed to interview the patient for 60 minutes, which is followed by a further 10 minutes to recollect thoughts and prepare for the interview with the examiners.

The actual clinical examination consists of:

10 minutes	for case presentation, including an assessment, which consists of salient features of the patient's aetiology, investigations, diagnosis, differential diagnosis, management and prognosis.
5–10 minutes	to interview the patient in the presence of the two examiners.
10–15 minutes	to discuss the case assessment in detail with the examiners.

These guidelines are divided into two parts:

(A) *Preparation for the examination:*

1. The examination is concerned with measuring your competency to manage patients with or without supervision.
2. There is no substitute for good clinical work and repeated practice with senior colleagues.
3. Ideally, the preparation should start from the day the examinee passes the MRCPsych Part I examination.

4. Be aware of common and uncommon diagnostic categories, their most important features, differential diagnosis and treatment aspects.

5. Practise on patients suffering from diseases in major diagnostic categories.

6. Develop a list of stock questions on major diagnostic categories.

7. Establish good understanding of ICD9, ICD10 (to be implemented in near future) or DSMIIIR.

8. Be aware of recent college reports, college statements, government papers and important articles in leading psychiatric and medical journals.

9. A thorough history taking and mental state examination will ensure that you do not miss the relevant issues in the case.

10. Be aware of legislative changes in the community care of psychiatric and elderly patients (NHS and Community Care Act 1990).

11. Making a correct diagnosis will not necessarily ensure that you pass the examination, but a critical appraisal of the patient's clinical problems is very important.

12. Practice will probably allow you to anticipate relevant questions in the examination.

(B) *Taking the clinical examination:*

1. Ask the patient by what name (i.e. surname or first name) you should address him or her.

2. Explain the purpose of the patient's involvement in the examination.

3. Introduce the patient to the examiners. Arrange chairs in a position which allows you good eye contact with the patient. At the end of the interview (in the presence of the examiners), see the patient off and thank him or her for cooperating.

4. During the 60-minute interview with the patient, start with open-ended and less demanding questions and work your way up. If you notice that the patient is getting irritable, impatient or annoyed, change the questions or take a break from your enquiry.

5. Pay due attention to the physical examination. It is no good saying that you did not have time to perform it. Be prepared to explain what you would be looking for in the patient; e.g. pulse, blood pressure, optic fundi, extra-pyramidal signs, thyroid gland, focal neurological signs, etc.

6. The examiners will remind you about the format of the examination. They may use various ways to ask you about the patient; e.g.

   'Tell us about your patient.'
   'Present your case.'
   'Give us the assessment of your patient.'
   'Give us a brief summary of your patient.'

7. Try to present your assessment from your memory rather than with constant reference to your handwritten notes.

8. Try to be confident and lucid.

9. Make use of relevant evidence from the literature to support your arguments.

10. The examiners will ask to explore or elicit a few relevant features of the patient's mental state, or the clinical history; e.g. obsessional features, mood, psychotic symptoms, thought content, insight, cognitive functions, premorbid personality, a typical drinking day, a typical anorexic/bulimic day, suicidal risk, etc. Occasionally, you may be asked to perform a brief neurological examination.

11. Write down the questions to be asked of the patient if you can't remember, as your anxiety level is likely to be high. If you do not understand any of the questions, ask the examiners to clarify them.

    The examiners are looking for therapeutic rapport, sensitivity and empathy, and will pose a selection of questions during the interview with the patient in their presence.

12. If you cannot reach a diagnosis, be prepared to discuss the case in terms of differential diagnosis in order of priority.

13. Try not to shoot yourself in the foot. Looking too anxious and nervous may result in an unwarranted disadvantage.

FURTHER READING

(A) Basic sciences

Psychology

1. Atkinson, R. L., Atkinson, R. C., Smith, E. and Bern, D. J. (1993) *Introduction to Psychology*, 11th edn, Orlando, FL: Harcourt Brace Jovanovich College Publishers.
2. Robbins, T. W. and Cooper, P. J. (1988) *Psychology for Medicine*, London: Edward Arnold.
3. Wolff, S. (1989) *Childhood and Human Nature: the Development of Personality*, London: Routledge.
4. Rust, J. and Golombok, S. (1989) *Modern Psychometrics: the Science of Psychological Assessment*, London: Routledge.

Sociology/social psychiatry

5. Fernando, S. (1989) *Race and Culture in Psychiatry*, London: Routledge.
6. Henderson, A. S. (1988) *An Introduction to Social Psychiatry*, New York: Oxford University Press.
7. Randall, F. and Wright, F. J. (1981) *Basic Sociology*, 4th edn, Plymouth: M & E Handbooks, Macdonald & Evans.

Basic psychodynamic concepts

8. Edelson, M. (1988) *Psychoanalysis: a Theory in Crisis*, Chicago: University of Chicago Press.

Neuroanatomy, neuropathology, neurophysiology, neurochemistry, psychopharmacology, genetics

9. Kendell, R. E. and Zealley, A. K. (eds) (1993) *Companion to Psychiatric Studies*, 5th edn, London: Churchill Livingstone.
10. Puri, B. K. and Tyrer, P. (1992) *Sciences Basic to Psychiatry*, Edinburgh: Churchill Livingstone.
11. Weller, M. and Eysenck, M. (eds) (1992) *The Scientific Basis of Psychiatry*, 2nd edn, London: W. B. Saunders Co. Ltd.

Psychopathology

12. Sims, A. (1991) *Symptoms in the Mind: an Introduction to Descriptive Psychopathology*, London: Baillière Tindall, W. B. Saunders.

Medical/psychiatric ethics

13. Bloch, S. and Chodoff, P. (eds) (1991) *Psychiatric Ethics*, 2nd edn, Oxford: Oxford Medical Publications, Oxford University Press.

Medical statistics

14. Bland, M. (1989) *An Introduction to Medical Statistics*, Oxford: Oxford University Press.
15. Bradford Hill, A. and Hall, I. D. (1991) *Bradford Hill's Medical Statistics*, 12th edn, London: Edward Arnold.

Research methodology

16. Freeman, C. and Tyrer, P. (eds) (1992) *Research Methods in Psychiatry: a Beginner's Guide*, 2nd edn, London: Gaskell, Royal College of Psychiatrists.

17. Thompson, C. (1989) *The Instruments of Psychiatric Research*, Chichester: Wiley.
18. Everitt, B. S. (1989) *Statistical Methods for Medical Investigations*, London: Edward Arnold.

(B) **Clinical psychiatry**

19. American Psychiatric Association (1987) *Diagnostic and Statistical Manual of Mental Disorders,* 3rd edn, revised (DSM-IIIR), Washington, DC: American Psychiatric Association.
20. Bancroft, J. (1989) *Human Sexuality and its Problems,* Edinburgh: Churchill Livingstone.
21. Bloch, S. (ed.) (1992) *An Introduction to the Psychotherapies*, 2nd edn, Oxford: Oxford Medical Publications, Oxford University Press.
22. Flach, F. (1989) *Psychotherapy*, London: W. W. Norton.
23. Gelder, M., Gath, D. and Mayou, R. (1989) *Oxford Textbook of Psychiatry*, 2nd edn, Oxford: Oxford Medical Publications, Oxford University Press.
24. Granville-Grossman, K. (ed.) (1993*) *Recent Advances in Psychiatry*, vols 1–8, Edinburgh: Churchill Livingstone.
25. Hill, P., Murray, R. and Thorley, A. (eds) (1989) *Essentials of Post Graduate Psychiatry*, London: Grune & Stratton.
26. Kaplan, I. and Sadock, J. (1991) *Synopsis of Psychiatry*, 6th edn, Baltimore, MD: Williams & Wilkins.
27. Kendell, R. E. and Zealley, A. K. (eds) (1993) *Companion to Psychiatric Studies*, 5th edn, London: Churchill Livingstone.
28. Lishman, A. (1987) *Organic Psychiatry: the Psychological Consequences of Cerebral Disorder*, 2nd edn, Oxford: Blackwell Scientific Publications.
29. Rutter, M. and Hersov, L. (eds) (1985) *Child and Adolescent Psychiatry: Modern Approaches*, 2nd edn, Oxford: Blackwell Scientific Publications.
30. World Health Organization (1992) *The ICD-10 Classification of Mental and Behavioural Disorders: Clinical Descriptions and Diagnostic Guidelines*, Geneva: World Health Organization.

*Date of the most recent volume

INDEX